32 MONDAYS

Weight Management Program

D1715651

WHAT ARANTXA'S CLIENTS HAVE TO SAY

I signed up for this program because I felt that my weight was out of control. Over the years, I kept buying larger clothes… It was really frustrating.

Arantxa understood very well the challenges of every step in my personal case, and was able to provide personalized solutions to increase my chance of success.

Arantxa helped me gain a much better understanding of the needs of the body and of the eating habits. Understanding of what and how to eat to keep the metabolism active helped me a lot and showed me why previous efforts failed.

Now I feel great because I can control when I eat, how much I eat, and what I eat. I feel in control of my weight again, and I know how to balance my diet and exercise. I was also able to lose more weight after I finished the 32 Mondays program.

—Jordi Tauler, Principal Scientific

I knew that knowledge about nutrition and exercise was the key to my long-term success. I signed up for the 32 Mondays program because I was confused by complicated food labels and marketing misconceptions of what exactly were the best foods and portion sizes for me.

During our sessions together and by following her website, Arantxa gave me confidence by explaining how different foods affect your body. She also taught me the most effective combination of eating and exercising.

With the knowledge I gained, I now feel empowered and in control of my weight. I am doing much better because of Arantxa's program, which I highly recommend to others who struggle with their weight.

—Kim Duffy, salon manager

I turned to Arantxa for help because I got frustrated with my weight. I wasn't able to lose it despite eating healthy and exercising!

Arantxa was able to identify my problem early on: I wasn't eating enough!

She explained to me why eating three meals a day and having snacks were important. I learned about the glycemic index and many other things that I had heard about before but didn't fully understand.

Arantxa was very supportive throughout the process, answering numerous questions…. It was enlightening to see how just a quick look at an ingredient list can help you make the right food choices.

I am happy to say that I achieved my goal weight. I look and feel great (just ask my husband)!

—Doris Guitelman, Realtor©

Arantxa helped me gain a much better understanding of how sugar and carbs affect my body by explaining short- and long-term effects. She also made me accountable for my actions by writing down what I ate each day so that I could be honest with myself.

Now I have much more knowledge about why I should stay away from certain foods and which food fuels my body with energy and health.

Arantxa also helped me select the right way to exercise to tone my body.

Weight loss is a journey, and I'm still on it! Arantxa gave me hope that I can do it.

—S. H., business owner

32 MONDAYS

Weight Management Program

An Educational Program to Manage Your Weight for Life

ARANTXA MATEO

ISBN 978-0-692-11534-3

The information and recommendations provided in the 32 Mondays Weight Management Program should never be considered a substitute for the advice of a qualified medical professional. This is especially important if you already suffer from an illness, are an aging person, or are pregnant or nursing.

Always consult a physician before beginning or changing your diet or exercise program, if you don't feel well, or if you experience a sudden change in your weight during the time you are following this program.

Publisher: Silver Note LLC

3 4015 07229 5643

This book is dedicated to my two daughters, Claudia and Greta, with the hope they become adults in a society with a healthy relationship with food.

In memory of my dog Luca, who left us in the middle of the writing of this book, who made me and my family happy for twelve and a half years, and who sat with me since the first day I started writing this book until his body couldn't handle it anymore.

I love you and miss you. Please wait for me at the Rainbow Bridge no matter how long it takes me to get there.

Luna, thank you for helping me overcome my grief and for sitting on my feet when I went back to writing.

CONTENTS

Preface xiii

Introduction. 1

Part I:

The 32 Mondays Weight Management Principles | 9

Principle 1: How The Program Works 11

Principle 2: Ditching The Diet Mentality. 19

Principle 3: Learning To Manage Your Weight 23

Principle 4: Learning To Take Control Of What You Eat 31

Principle 5: Mastering Grocery Shopping. 39

Principle 6: Navigating The Kitchen. 45

Principle 7: Physical And Psychological Food Addictions 51

Principle 8: All About Insulin. 57

Principle 9: Learning About Other Hormones 67

Principle 10: Understanding Metabolic Syndrome 75

Part II:

32 Mondays Weight Management Program's 15 Steps | 81

Step 1: Eat Less Every Meal 83

Step 2: Start Moderate Exercise 91

Step 3: Drinks 101

Step 4: Composition And Organization Of Meals 111

Step 5: Snacking. 129

Step 6: Fats 137

Step 7: Sugars. 147

Step 8: Carbohydrates 157

Step 9: Salt. 163

Step 10: Alcohol. 167

Step 11: Vigorous Exercise 171

Step 12: Fruits And Vegetables 187

Step 13: Sleep. 193

Step 14: Go Organic 197

Step 15: Be Happy For The Rest Of Your Life 209

Part III
Additional Information | 215

Acknowledgments 223

Appendix A: Recommended Resources. 225

Appendix B: Height / Weight / Bmi Chart And Waist Circumference
    Values 227

Appendix C: Calories Burned When Exercising 231

Appendix D: List Of Sugar Names 233

Appendix E: Grocery Store Shopping List 237

Appendix F: Weekly Meal Plan 241

Food Journal Template. 250

About The Author 253

Index 255

Notes 259

PREFACE

This book is not about a diet. Instead, it describes a process. It is a process to change your relationship with food. It is structured into steps, and every step will give you time to master it before moving onto the next one. By the time you have gone through all the steps, you'll be a new you.

I am not talking only about weight management but also about health improvement. Let's be honest: improvement of our self-image is the first thing we are all looking for. A positive self-image doesn't mean you need to look perfect, but at least you have to like yourself. Don't hide behind the idea of "Being fat is as cool as being thin." We know this is not true. I watched an interview with an actress who spoke about how well she felt after losing an impressive amount of weight, yet months ago she had also appeared on TV stating how important it was for her to feel okay with her own body even knowing she was overweight. Within a few months she had made totally contradictory declarations; which one do you think was the sincere one?

We like ourselves better when we look great. This is reality, whether we want to admit it or not. This is the main trigger and motivator for changing the way we eat.

When I was at university studying for my biology degree, I had a close friend who studied to become a physical education teacher/sports trainer. He asked me why I liked swimming so much; I told him because it was good for my back and my health, and it made me feel relaxed after studying for long hours. He disputed that and told me: "Face it. The truth is you like swim-ming because you like how it shapes your body." Back then I was too young to admit that. In retrospect, I know he was right. Now that I am older I keep swimming for both reasons. Swimming is really healthy, and it does wonders for my back, but it is true that a big motivator to keep swimming is that it still keeps my body in good shape.

> *Improving the way you see yourself is the first health benefit you'll notice. The health of your mind has a lot to do with the health of your body.*

In my opinion, the first negative health effect of being overweight is the psychological one, and you don't even need to be highly overweight to feel the effect in your mind. **When you are not at peace with your body, you don't feel good about yourself.** When you have a negative relationship with your inner self, your physical health can be affected, and a vicious circle begins: the less you like yourself, the less you care. This is an indirect health effect of being overweight, as powerful as a "direct" effect.

You probably already know most of the direct health risks associated with bad eating habits, with being overweight. But a quick reminder won't hurt; these include:

> › depression

> › type 2 diabetes

> › atherosclerosis (hardening of the arteries)

> › stroke

> › high blood pressure

> › high cholesterol

> › higher risk of heart attack

> › several types of cancer (colon, kidney, digestive tract, and other)

> › overstressed and painful joints

> arthritis

> mental well-being

> breathing problems

> heartburn

Chances are if you are overweight, you don't exercise enough either, so add the negative health effects of not exercising enough: lack of energy; low level of endorphins; lower flexibility; lower organ and cell oxygenation; compromised lung and heart function. You don't need to have all of those conditions to make your life miserable and even cut your life expectancy drastically. **You only need one of those conditions to really have to worry about your health and your quality of life and your future.**

You might be someone who is at your ideal right weight and happy with it, but who struggles every day to keep it that way. The 32 Mondays Weight Management Program is also for you. You can't struggle all your life to keep your weight down, always obsessed with what you eat to avoid gaining an inch or centimeter and/or killing yourself in the gym to keep your weight where it needs to be. Don't you see this can keep you in a constant bad mood and inhibit you from enjoying life? Yes, it is possible to maintain your weight by following a more rational way of eating and exercising.

Food is a pleasure. We all deserve to enjoy food. But we need to re-educate our taste away from what the food industry has manipulated and relearn how to enjoy healthy foods. That is the focus of the 32 Mondays Weight Management Program.

INTRODUCTION

When I was the age my daughters are now, we didn't know too much about nutrition and its relationship to our health and the way we eat. Basically, our approach when it came to food was, "I like it or I don't like it," or "It is good for me or it isn't." Maybe we had a general idea of the benefits of fruits and vegetables. However, if you were lucky, as I was, you had a mom who was interested in health and nutrition—back then, dads didn't have much to do with their kids, let alone their nutrition—and maybe she considered nutrition a core part of a kid's development. Perhaps she even looked for a pediatrician with similar beliefs.

As I said, I had one of those moms. My diet and nutrition were quite good. On the other hand, I grew up in Spain, a country that had a civil war when my parents were young, and they lived through a famine associated with the aftermath of that war. As a result, when I was a kid—and even though the war had been over for more than thirty years—parents still felt it was important to have enough food, and they tended to overfeed their kids. Ours was also a society that was not used to exercise (although we loved to watch sports on TV), and my family was no exception. By the time I was six years old, I was a little bit overweight, and the negative way I saw myself and how bad I felt at school grew with each year. By the time I was ten, my parents were divorced. I spent long hours at home alone while my mom worked two nursing shifts, night and morning. I learned to overindulge myself with potato chips, ice cream, and sandwiches, which you could already see in my figure and consequently, in my self-esteem.

By fourteen, during the summer before high school, I was quite mature and independent, and I decided I didn't want to be overweight anymore. I wanted a new me. I wanted a new image for myself to start this new chapter of my life in high school. That summer I started to lose a lot of weight by just eating less. I don't remember ever being hungry, just eating less.

I was a freshman in high school when I had a lesson on nutrition, and this is where I learned about calories, vitamins, and minerals. That marked a point of no return in my life. I became so interested in the concept of nutrition, and more specifically weight management, that it became one of my priorities and main interests. Basically, I didn't want to ever get overweight again, so I wanted to learn all the specifics about how what you eat (your nutrition) affects your weight, and how, with the right information, it is easy to avoid weight gain (weight management).

That year I started to learn how to cook. I would eat lunch at home by myself, and I had to cook what my mom left for me. I learned that instead of fried chicken, I would rather have grilled chicken. I didn't need fried croutons in my vegetable puree. Coffee without sugar was cool, and everything could be cooked or baked with less fat and sugar.

By my second year in high school, I was a skinny teenager. I have to admit my mother suffered at some points thinking I was close to anorexia, but I wasn't. I just realized I didn't need to eat so much and I would rather eat healthy food that made me feel good. I also discovered the physical and mental benefits of exercise. I have followed those principles to this day.

I hold a degree in biology, which I earned in Spain (where you have to study five years of pure and strict science). After three years of more general subjects like physics, math, chemistry, biochemistry, genetics, microbiology, animal and vegetal physiology, and related subjects, you choose your specialty. In my case, as a practical and hands-on woman, I decided I wanted a practical subject. So I specialized in applied biology, including nutrition biochemistry. My specialty gave me tools and the ability to understand life science-related problems and solutions. Over the years, and after additional studies and professional experience, I have applied this ability to many things, but it has been as a weight management mentor that I have discovered what I was always meant to be.

Since that time almost twenty years ago, the amount of available information on nutrition has increased exponentially. We now know so much about the biochemistry of food, the way our metabolism processes it, how our hormones are related to our weight management, and more, that you would think society's nutrition has improved in the same way as scientific knowledge. But the reality is that it hasn't happened this way. We could even say some people are worse off now in terms of their relationship with food, the way it nourishes their bodies and contributes to weight gain. Others have been fighting to manage their weight management their entire lives—and losing, probably because of misinformation and lack of adequate education. Even people who maintain the right weight still struggle to get skinnier in order to fit into the new silhouette stereotype.

Something is not right. We have more and more information but are getting worse results. Society has changed in other aspects, too. We work long hours. More women are in the labor force and struggling to balance work and family. We don't have time to shop for our groceries and cook healthy meals, let alone learn the latest on nutrition and weight management, and little time to exercise.

In the meantime, more "miracle" diets come to life. Most of the diets are totally contradictory, and this adds still more confusion into our lives. When yesterday the advice was a fat-free diet, today it is high fat and low carbohydrates, or high protein and low carbohydrates. Or it is vegetarianism or even no fruits or vegetables. Or eat all you want, but only if it is green. Or count every calorie you put into your mouth. Or starve yourself. Or exercise until exhaustion. Or motivate yourself by telling yourself you are a loser if you are fat. Or insult yourself because you love certain foods. I think I have heard everything, but I am still surprised when a new version of a "diet" appears.

Some people are quite successful on these diets for a short time, but most people usually gain back some or all their lost weight on most of them. For some other people it takes longer to recover the lost weight, but they will eventually regain much of it.

Most diets are based on giving you a solution to your problem. You can hear kids saying, "I want it, and I want it now!" We are not too different from them; we have a problem, and we want a solution… and if possible, we want that solution without too much effort or too much thinking. So that is what we get with most diets: an eating "plan" based on some general principles that might sound more or less correct, and a list of what to eat each day so we don't have to think too much. This works for a while for people who are able to follow the rules, but it doesn't work anymore once we are left on our own: we get distracted, we lose our motivation, we forget some of the steps, we hate being on a diet, we didn't buy the right ingredients … and so on and so on.

You can't be on a diet all of your life. You can't live every day starving for food. You can't go and buy exactly what you need for your recipe and for your dinner every night if you don't have enough time. You can't eat what you don't like. You can't avoid everything you do like. You can't follow directions if you don't understand what you are doing, or expect to be able to repeat the steps on your own once you don't have that direction.

With all the advances in the science of nutrition and weight management, there should be a better approach to healthy living than a simple diet.

I am convinced of the power of knowledge and education. We spend long hours and thousands of dollars on our children's education and even on our own education. But we don't value the importance of nutrition and weight management education, even when that knowledge will influence how we live and our future quality of life. We simply don't know enough, and we have misconceptions.

Balance in your diet is the main concept of the 32 Mondays Weight Management Program. You'll find plenty of books discussing the pros and cons of the most famous diets—high/low fat, protein, carbohydrate, and others—if you want to know more, but those are not the focus of this book.

In this book, I want to educate—or in most cases, re-educate—you about the way you eat and how to be weight managers and health improvers. Since most of you don't have a lot of time, I have created a simple and structured Program that is easy to follow and learn, and therefore simple to maintain for life.

My goal is to instill good eating habits in you and in the society in which my daughters will grow and live.

ᣞ

The 32 Mondays Weight Management Program is a way of life, not a diet. It is a step-by-step process that will systematically change your relationship with food and will teach you how to gain control of your weight for the rest of your life.

You will feel so good while following the Program that you will start every Monday invigorated and ready to learn and apply all the new concepts every one to three weeks, depending on where you are in the Program and how much you already know or need to modify your habits. This is why the Program is called 32 Mondays: for thirty-two weeks, you'll embrace this Program full of energy, which will lead you to finally gain control of your weight management for life.

ᣞ

This book is structured into three parts:

Part I introduces the 10 Principles of the 32 Mondays Weight Management Program. These are the basics you need to know and understand for optimum weight loss and to make the changes I'll be asking you to make in your habits. At the end of each Principle you will find a summary of key points, which you can refer to as needed as you work your way through the Program.

Part II introduces each of the 15 Steps of the Program. Each chapter gives detailed information about a particular step and how to master it in practice. For every step, there is a recommendation for the number of weeks I suggest you dedicate to mastering that step before moving on. Please note that each step builds on the previous one, and you may be practicing multiple steps simultaneously. After completing the number of weeks recommended in each step, you will have mastered the Program in *32 Mondays*. Depending on your previous knowledge and your starting point, you might need less time to finish the whole Program, but make sure you give yourself enough time to learn, practice, and interiorize (or even change) new or (inadequate) habits.

At the end of each Step, you will find a "Take 5" section, where I'll ask you to:

> › learn

> › set goals

> › plan

> › monitor, and

> › get a reward

for each of the steps. This is important because each of those five aspects are essential to succeed in this Program. Please, pay attention to them and make sure you do them.

I recommend you read all the steps once before you start the Program so you familiarize yourself with each of them. Many of them are related, and it might be difficult to understand them if you don't have the whole picture.

Finally, **in Part III you will find other information that might be of interest**: kids and healthy eating, and supplements and pharmaceuticals. And don't miss the appendices, which contain recommended resources, a food journal, and more.

෨

Please visit my website at *32Mondays.com* for more information. While you're there, don't forget to register for my newsletter to get fresh news, tips, and ideas every week. And if you ever have doubts or need to clarify something, feel free to send me an email at arantxamateo@32mondays.com.

The journey you are beginning is not an easy one. You have probably tried many times in the past to lose weight by enrolling in programs or following different diets, and you've probably spent some money along the way. If you are reading this book now, it is because whatever you have tried in the past hasn't worked for you; either you weren't successful in losing weight, you gained back the weight, or maintaining your weight was so difficult that you want to find a better way.

I can't tell you my way is an easy way. Any change in habits requires an effort and a change of mind-set that might take you some time and effort.

But what I can tell you is that the Program I am offering will not make you feel hungry, tired, or miserable. I am going to show you the way to gain control over your weight management so you feel empowered and satisfied with the results you get when you invest the time, effort, and dedication to understand and follow the 32 Mondays Program.

The changes you are about to make will fill you with energy and satisfaction, which will help you to keep going and feel still better one step at a time.

Because the Program is so structured and well planned, you won't feel lost or left on your own. I'll be there guiding you through each step until you master it and can move to the next one, and eventually master the entire 32 Mondays Program. I will guide you through a journey that will allow you to finally gain control of your weight and consequently feel better, with more energy and confidence, and, most important, be healthier.

Nobody can take this journey for you, and it is probably the most rewarding one you'll ever take. One thing I know about weight management is this: if you keep doing the same thing day after day and month after month, you will continue to get similar results. No change means no progress. If you don't do anything right now, tomorrow you will wake up the same. Only you can decide when it's time to change your life. So please, jump with me into the 32 Mondays Weight Loss Program, and let me help you discover a new you.

PART I

THE 32 MONDAYS WEIGHT MANAGEMENT PRINCIPLES

Part I will explain the principles you need to know and understand to learn and master the 32 Mondays Weight Management Program.

Here you will learn how the Program is structured and will find tips to help you succeed. We will talk about weight management, what it means, and how to determine your perfect weight. You will also learn how to develop the right attitude for success. To do so, you will need to know how to master grocery store shopping and how to navigate your kitchen—at least a little bit. Finally, we'll discuss physical and psychological food addictions, and you'll learn about managing insulin and other hormone levels and look at the condition called metabolic syndrome—a cluster of the most dangerous heart attack risk facts: diabetes, abdominal obesity, high (bad) cholesterol, and high blood pressure. Armed with this information, you'll understand and recognize what happens in your body when you eat certain foods and engage in certain eating behaviors.

Please read all the principles as many times as you need to fully comprehend them and to help you understand the method. Here they are again:

✌

Principle 1: How the Program Works

Principle 2: Ditching the Diet Mentality

Principle 3: Learning to Manage Your Weight

Principle 4: Learning to Take Control of What You Eat

Principle 5: Mastering Grocery Shopping

Principle 6: Navigating the Kitchen

Principle 7: Physical and Psychological Food Addictions

Principle 8: All about Insulin

Principle 9: Learning about Other Hormones

Principle 10: Understanding Metabolic Syndrome

PRINCIPLE 1
HOW THE PROGRAM WORKS

The 32 Mondays Weight Management Program will teach you how to eat appropriately, have an active lifestyle, and maintain your weight loss—forever. This structured method uses a step-by-step approach that helps you easily learn and assimilate all the skills you need to succeed and maintain your weight for the rest of your life. This is *not* a temporary diet you use until you fit into your old dress, feel comfortable in a bikini, or get married. It's a change in the way you feed and exercise your body for the rest of your life.

The Program consists of fifteen steps. Each step is designed to help you master one aspect of losing weight, maintaining weight, changing how you eat, bolstering your nutrition, taking control of your diet, and adding exercise to your daily life. Every step comes with a recommendation for how many weeks you will need to master that step, consolidate its concepts, and move on to the next step.

You can't start learning the next step until the previous one has been mastered and incorporated into your way of living. Each step then becomes a habit, something you do without even thinking about it. You will then move to the next step until you master that one, too, and so on.

When you add up all the weeks recommended for each step, you will see that it takes you thirty-two weeks to master all the steps and therefore incorporate the entire 32 Mondays Weight Management Program forever.

Every step has its own challenges. Some steps are more difficult than others. I have allowed a specific number of weeks for each step depending on the difficulty I think you might encounter before you are able to master it.

The Program has been designed to guide you through different changes in the way you eat, drink, exercise, and live. It will help you transform what and when you eat and drink, and how you exercise, sleep, and organize your meals.

Every step in this method has a specific reason for being included, and all of them are interrelated. Our bodies are complex organisms. Whatever happens in one part of us is related to or has consequences in other parts. Your nutrition and your way of living greatly affect how your body works. The 32 Mondays Weight Management Program will teach you the best and easiest ways to manage all the internal aspects related to your weight management (hormone release, brain signals, and so on) by controlling how you do things on the outside—eat, move, sleep, and the like.

Each person will feel differently about each step. Some people will struggle with eliminating or modifying a certain habit while others may have already done so. We are all different, with different feelings, attachments, preferences, attitudes, expectations, desires, and readiness. That is why a diet or a method generalized for everybody is a difficult fit for us as individuals. We need a personalized system designed for who we are. The only person who can really master that method is you.

As I said before, if you apply my time line recommendations for each step, it will take you 32 Mondays to master this Program. Each step lasts for a specific number of weeks for a reason. Following the Program time line is important because you need deadlines, target dates, and challenges to achieve your goals. If you leave the time line open, you will be tempted to sit back and relax, and time will pass without you making progress. Keep to the defined number of weeks, and if you haven't mastered a step, keep practicing its principles while starting the next step.

This doesn't mean it will take you thirty-two weeks to lose all the weight you want to lose. It means that after thirty-two weeks, you will have mastered the method and therefore will be able to stay focused on continuing to lose weight until you reach your perfect weight. More important, once you have mastered this Program, you will be able to maintain that weight easily with no extra effort.

And down the line, if you deviate from your ideal weight and need to lose some extra weight (for example, after a special occasion or a celebration), you will have learned from this method how to put in the extra effort to lose that weight: by cutting the size of your meals a bit more, by cutting out all your treats for a while, or by cutting back again on sugars and carbohydrates.

Remember: this is *not* a diet. This is an educational program to learn how, when, and what to eat; how to cook, shop, and exercise. Your goal is to be able to manage your optimal weight forever.

The objective is to concentrate on one specific step at a time. Invest all your energy on only one step. Once you have mastered that specific step, you will move on to concentrate on the next one. You will have imbedded the old one in your brain and assimilated it into your behavior. You don't have a great deal of surplus energy to manage juggling three or four major tasks at a time. You need to make these life changes as easy as possible. That is why the objective here is to concentrate on *only* one step at a time.

There are fifteen steps to be mastered in Thirty-two weeks. You can do that!

Monitoring Your Weight, Food Intake, Exercise, and Sleep: A Special Note

Monitoring weight, food intake, exercise, and sleep is a critical aspect of this Program if you want to succeed. I am going to ask you to monitor your weight, keep a food, exercise, and sleep journal, and plan and follow menus.

Monitor Your Weight

By monitoring your weight weekly (at least during the next thirty-two weeks), you will be able to follow objectively how you are losing weight step-by-step. Once you are at your desired weight, I will ask you to monitor your weight almost every day to make sure you are maintaining your weight and not gaining weight without realizing it.

Food, Exercise, and Sleep Journal

I recommend you keep the journal at least until you have completed the 32 Mondays Weight Management Program. By keeping a food, exercise, and sleep diary, you will know how much you are actually eating, drinking, exercising, and sleeping. That way you will be able to look back and pinpoint what can be cut and what can be changed. Your journal will be a tremendous help for learning about yourself and setting specific goals for each step.

You will be tracking two types of progress:

› Daily progress. The first reason is that by nighttime, you'll probably have already forgotten what you ate in the morning, and it is important to know exactly what and how much is going into your mouth so you can make sure you are really following the recommendations of each step.

› Overall progress. The second reason to keep a food journal is to use it as a reference and to record your overall progress. By reviewing your journal, you'll be able to know how you have changed your eating, activity, and sleeping habits. You will also see how much healthier you are feeling, and that will reinforce what you are doing. The Food and Exercise Journal will also be helpful when you slip from the right path, which will happen from time to time. It will help you look back and see how much you have accomplished since you started so you will be motivated to keep going instead of throwing in the towel.

Keep a journal that best fits you. In Appendix G, you will find an example of a food journal that you can also use as a sleep and exercise journal. You can always use something as simple as a notebook or something as sophisticated as a phone app to track your food, sleep, and exercise—*whatever works best for you is the best method.* List what and how much you eat—*everything*—and how much you exercise—moderate or vigorous—and how much you sleep. If you Google *food journal* or *food diary*, you will find many examples, web pages, apps, and other tools that can help you decide which is the right one for you.

Follow a Menu Plan

Given our busy lifestyles, it is not surprising that we often struggle to make good decisions and think clearly by the end of the day. When you get home hungry and exhausted from your day-to-day activities, which often include making tough decisions, you don't have too much energy left over to decide what to eat for dinner or what to prepare for the next day's lunch. That's why you need to plan ahead and know exactly what you are going to eat without having to think about it. That means having a menu planner, which lets you know what groceries you need and when you can find time to cook, or when to prepare the meals ahead of time and then store them to be used when you don't have time to prepare them. Remember this: the more you plan your weekly meals, the more you will succeed.

Unless you were pregnant or had an upsetting event in your life, it is unlikely you gained your extra weight in just a few days. It took you months and years to get where you are. You can't expect to lose that extra weight in just a few days!

When you follow the 32 Mondays Weight Management Program, you will see a steady weight loss over time. The more you need to lose, the quicker you'll see the results. Once you are close to your optimal weight, losing weight will become more difficult and slower. If you choose to go beyond your ideal weight, it will get hard, and you will need to make a significant sacrifice to keep losing that additional weight.

The 32 Mondays Weight Management Program includes basic recommendations, like eating less, and practical ones, like how to plan for buying the appropriate groceries. It also goes into the technical aspects of weight management—for example, how the hormone insulin works—and more down-to-earth recommendations, like how to cook. The entire method is a learning process, so you will understand what to eat and how to find recipes that you and your family like and are easy for you to prepare. By the end of the book, you will know how to plan what to eat and how to cook or prepare it for each meal. Every new step will start by reminding you about the previous step and reinforcing the concepts you have learned to make sure you have naturally incorporated them into your way of eating and living.

I know we are talking about hard work. I am going to ask you to make many changes, including how you shop at your grocery store. You'll begin to plan meals, cook, keep food journals, and do many other things you might not be doing right now. But we are talking about changing habits and unhealthy conditions that took you years to develop. Yes, it is hard work, but it is a lifetime investment to undo years of bad habits. Keep in mind how much energy and time-consuming it is for a diabetic to check his/her blood sugar levels daily and to manage his/her medication. The same is true with hypertension and other diseases that develop as a result of poor nourishment. Come on! Wouldn't you rather invest your time to learn the 32 Mondays Weight Management Program and be healthy *forever* than invest your time to take care of yourself once you are sick?

The Take 5 Approach

The Take 5 approach is widely used as a risk management tool in the health, safety, and environmental industries. The core idea is to encourage you to think before acting—that is, to take some time before acting to help you to stop, observe, think, decide, and plan an action whenever you are confronted with an unusual and potentially unsafe situation. It is a concept I have always loved, and I have decided to adapt the Take 5 idea as the basis for following the 32 Mondays Weight Management Program.

It might be a good idea to write down the Take 5 for each step in your journal so you can see it while following the step. In each step, it is important to:

1. **LEARN** what to do in each step by taking the time to read and understand the information included in each chapter.

2. **SET GOALS** so you have a specific objective.

3. **PLAN** how you will accomplish each step. Things don't just happen. You have to *make* them happen.

4. **MONITOR** your results and hold yourself accountable for your changes.

5. **REWARD** your effort and commitment each time you accomplish a new step.

KEY POINTS

This is an educational program composed of fifteen steps that are to be mastered in thirty-two weeks. Follow the program step-by-step until each one is mastered, and remember these key points:

- › Monitoring and planning are essential.
  - ○ Weigh yourself and keep records.
  - ○ Maintain a food, exercise, and sleep journal.
  - ○ Menu planning will keep you on track.
- › Miracle diets fail and quick fixes don't work. Take your time.
- › Follow the Take 5 approach:
  - ○ Learn
  - ○ Set Goals
  - ○ Plan
  - ○ Monitor
- › Reward

PRINCIPLE 2
DITCHING THE DIET MENTALITY

This weight management program is not a diet. Instead, it includes basic recommendations like eating less, to practical ones like how to buy the appropriate groceries. It also goes into the technical aspects of weight management—for example: "How does the hormone insulin work?" and more down-to-earth recommendations like how to cook. The entire method is a learning process, so I am not telling you exactly what to eat and I am not giving you a recipe for every meal. By the end of the book, you will know how to plan what to eat and how to cook or prepare it for each meal. Every new step will start reminding you about the previous step and reinforcing the concepts you have learned, to make sure you have naturally incorporated them into your mind and your way of eating and living.

Why Miracle Diets Fail and Quick Fixes Don't Work

Everybody wants a quick fix. Just a few changes without too much effort and… voilà, in just a short time, you have a new weight and a new life—forever. The reality is that a quick fix doesn't exist. When you find a diet that makes you lose a lot of weight in a short period of time, it doesn't come cheap in terms of your long-term health. It either asks you to significantly restrict the number of calories you are ingesting, accompanied by the significant effort that it takes and the subsequent tiring results, or it bans an important and necessary group of nutrients for a certain period of time—either protein, fats, or carbohydrates. In this second scenario, you usually lose weight because the eating process gets so boring that you end up eating less.

In both scenarios, sooner or later you end up regaining most of the weight you lost. In the first scenario, after suppressing the amount of calories you ingest, your body starts to economize its energy expenditure, using less calories than before for the same activities, and it learns how to use the limited energy available as efficiently as possible. When you return to a higher calorie intake, your body will be able to spend less energy for daily activities and will use the energy more efficiently, making you recover the lost weight and gain even more; **this is the yo-yo effect of dieting.** You will also lose muscle mass in the process. You will learn later how muscle helps you burn calories and therefore maintain your weight. In the second scenario, when you are done with your miracle diet and are allowed to introduce more of a variety of ingredients after restricting a certain group of foods, you tend to overeat them because you have missed those foods so much!

Yo-Yo Dieting: A Special Note

Yo-yo dieting is the result of a calorie-restrictive diet. Your body gets used to spending less energy for basic processes, which is called lowering your metabolism. When you go back to a higher calorie intake, your body will still use less energy, and it will save as much energy as possible as fat, in case the calorie availability is reduced in the future. As a result, you gain weight easily just from taking in some extra calories.

If you have just been in a calorie restrictive diet, you probably have lost significant muscle mass during the process. When you are on a diet that restricts calorie intake, your body turns to burning muscle to obtain sugar from protein and feed the brain (which eats only sugars) and lowers metabolism to get the maximum outcome with the lowest calorie intake. **Yo-yo dieting leaves you with less muscle (your ally to burn calories) and a lower metabolic rate (your calorie burner).** It will take a while to reactivate your metabolism, but you will get there once you are following the 32 Mondays Weight Management Program.

Food Lovers

We all love food. We are born with the natural ability to love food to be able to survive. If babies didn't like eating, they would die. But a big part of the eating process is education. Depending on how you educate your taste buds, you are going to like a specific type of food more or less. This is the part you can manage to get in control of your weight. By cooking the foods you like and that are good for you in an appropriate way, you will reeducate your own taste buds until you begin to crave the right food for you.

There are people who only eat to survive and who do not derive any pleasure or satisfaction from the process of eating, and they only eat to have enough energy to keep going. But if you investigate a little, you'll find that most of them had a poor education in relation to food and eating. Most of them come from families who never enjoyed the pleasure of a good meal, especially together.

There are other people who do like food and enjoy eating but who are slaves of their self-image and never see themselves as thin enough, so they perpetually starve themselves. You can recognize them easily. They are those skinny ladies (or men) who always wear a bitter expression in their faces. Who can blame them? How can you be happy if you are never satisfied enough with yourself and your body, if you're continuously hungry, and if you never freely enjoy a tasty meal without feeling guilty? This is the fault of poor information. If you knew better, you would learn first that it is not natural to be below your optimal weight; your body fights to recover the weight. The body reacts to being underweight by extracting as much energy as possible from anything consumed and at the same time expending as little energy (calories) as possible. Once you know more, you can keep almost the same weight by simply changing the way you eat with no need to starve.

My family is made up of food lovers. I once asked my aunt why was it that our family life always revolved around the kitchen and food. She answered me that it was a way to communicate love for each other, by cooking and sharing the food with love. I have to say that my family's ancestors were all poor communicators in expressing their feelings, so they probably had to find a new and effective way to communicate love.

So let's ditch crash dieting and enjoy food!

Enjoying Sweet Treats Responsibly

Most of us like to have sweet treats, and we either overdo them or are constantly depriving ourselves of them. It is okay to have a daily treat, but we need a few considerations:

› Make sure you treat yourself only once a day, and try to leave it for the end of the day.

› Eat your treat at the end of the meal to avoid glucose and insulin peaks.

› Have a treat that's as healthy as possible: dark chocolate is better than milk chocolate, homemade or organic cookies are better than packaged ones, or a few organic chocolate-covered nuts instead of a candy bar.

KEY POINTS

› The 32 Mondays Weight Management Program is not a diet.

› Diets do not work.

› Avoid yo-yo dieting.

› It is healthy to love food; educate yourself.

› Enjoy sweet treats responsibly.

PRINCIPLE 3
LEARNING TO MANAGE YOUR WEIGHT

You are going to learn what "weight management" really means. You will also learn what reference measures you can use to evaluate where you are now, and how you can determine your perfect weight. Those values will help you address your weight management.

Weight management is not only about weight, it is also about how you feel and see yourself. You should learn to enjoy the feeling of physical and psychological improvement. This improvement is what you get when you manage your weight appropriately. I know it sounds kind of esoteric, but you will understand better once you start following the 32 Mondays Weight Management Program. In the meantime, let's move to more practical matters to help you determine where you are now in terms of your weight by using some **reference measures** to help you find an **overall evaluation** of your weight.

> The journey between where you are and where you should be and how you maintain it once you're there is what I call Weight Management.

Monitoring Weight Effectively

During the initial weight loss period, you should avoid checking your weight obsessively. When you use the scale, no matter how often you do, you always end up stressed, so no stepping onto the scale several times a day or after each workout. **While you are in the process of losing weight, you should use weight only as an additional indicator once a week to help you monitor your results.**

How much you actually weigh is debatable. It depends on what hour of the day you weigh yourself, how much water you are retaining at that specific moment, what you ate last week, and even what you had for dinner the night before. Your weight will also be affected if you are suffering from stress or you are at peace with yourself. There are so many variables affecting your weight at any specific moment that it makes weight a controversial measure of health. Obviously, it is important to know your weight at specific times, such as when you need to start on medication or modify its dosage. You also need to determine your weight if you are going to undergo surgery or when you see an important change in your health. But weight on its own is not a good measure for evaluating how you are doing in terms of your body shape management.

The problem of using only weight as a reference is that you obsess about it when you don't see an important decrease over a certain period of time. You think you are failing, your morale decreases, and you lose focus and control. You will certainly see you are losing weight even if you don't use the scale too often. Check how your clothing fits and measure your waist circumference. You might be losing inches everywhere while your weight initially stays the same. This is because you are losing fat and gaining muscle, and the fat weighs less than the muscle, so there is no change in total weight. This is really evident after you start having a more active life. Remember: this is a learning Program, and it will take you a while to learn a new way to eat and integrate a new lifestyle before you start to lose weight consistently.

Once you have seen and felt significant weight loss, you can start checking your weight on the scale more often to keep track and monitor your progress. Once you achieve your desired weight, you can use the scale several times a week or even daily. By monitoring your weight closely, you can act as soon as you see a deviation from your ideal weight and never allow the extra weight to stay for too long.

If you are able to:

› avoid obsessing about your weight,

› accept that even if your weight is staying the same, you might be changing your body composition for good, and

› recognize that weight fluctuates a lot from one day to the next for many reasons—these include more or less sleep, how much salty food you consumed, and how tired you are—

then you should follow these recommendations to keep track of how are you doing:

› weigh once a week during the initial period;

› weigh several times a week once you have lost considerable weight; and

› weigh almost every day during the maintenance period.

If weighing yourself creates too much anxiety, wait to use the scale until you are several weeks into the program, when you can already see some changes in your body shape.

Reference Measures

Aside from weekly weight measurement, I like to use two indicators as a reference to evaluate where you are in terms of health and to evaluate improvement. Those reference measures are called **body mass index (BMI)** and **waist circumference**. According to the International Diabetes Federation (IDF), a healthy person in North America will have a BMI value below 25 to 29, and a waist circumference below 40.16 inches (102 cm) for males and 34.65 inches (88 cm) for females.[1] It is interesting to note that the values for Europeans and all other ethnic groups are way below those for people in the United States. Are overweight Americans with more abdominal fat/circumference "normal"?

Where do you fit in? Calculate your own BMI and waist circumference after reading the sections below.

Body Mass Index (BMI)

BMI is a measure based on height and weight. It is the measurement used by doctors to assess whether a person has an appropriate weight or is overweight or even obese based on his/her height and weight.

Its main limitation is it doesn't consider that muscle mass weighs much more than fat. So if you have a muscular constitution, you may actually have a higher BMI than someone with more fat. Some athletes' BMI falls into the overweight classification even though they are clearly not overweight. Their constitution of lean body mass, with lots of muscle and little fat, gives them a higher BMI than a "normal" person. If your muscle mass is greater than average, you should take this limitation into consideration when calculating your BMI.

To calculate your BMI:

BMI = (weight in pounds) / (height in inches)^2) x 703

or

BMI = (weight in grams) / (height in meters)^2

Body Mass Index	Category
Below 18.5	Underweight
18.5–24.9	Healthy weight
25.0–29.9	Overweight
30–30.9	Obese
Over 40	Morbidly obese

For example, a man of five feet six inches, whose weight is 175 pounds (or 167.6 cm and 79.4 kg):

BMI= ((175)/(66x66)) x 703 = (175/4356) x 703= 28.24

He will be overweight.

A woman of five feet three inches whose weight is 172 pounds (or 160 cm and 78 kg):

BMI: 78,000/(1.6) x (1.60) = 78,000/256 = 30.47

She will be entering into obesity.[2]

See Appendix B to determine your maximum weight based on your height according to your BMI, or find a BMI calculator online.

WAIST CIRCUMFERENCE

Excess body fat in the abdomen, measured as waist circumference, is the most unhealthy and dangerous fat in your body. A prominent belly signals fat accumulation in the abdominal area around your vital organs (visceral fat in the stomach, liver, and intestines). Those organs suffer the consequences of having all that fat around—more bad fat in the blood is carried to those organs, and therefore more fat accumulation. A person with high volumes of abdominal fat also produces hormones that create an imbalance in their metabolic equilibrium. This imbalance increases the risk of heart attack, breathing problems, certain types of cancer, stroke, hypertension, cholesterol, diabetes, and related issues. In terms of health, reduction of waist circumference needs to be your main focus. It is not by chance that when the IDF achieved a worldwide consensus for the definition of metabolic syndrome in 2006, it used central obesity—body fat in the abdomen—as one of the causes, and used waist circumference as one of the tools to assess the risk of a person suffering metabolic syndrome. (You'll learn more about metabolic syndrome in Principle 10.)

A Note of Caution

When you start to change your diet and begin a moderate exercise program, you may initially substitute fat for muscle. Even though you will be losing fat, your BMI and weight may not only remain the same, they could even rise. This is because muscle weighs more than fat, so you'll weigh more. You have to be cautious when interpreting your improvement. If you think you are truly substituting fat for muscle, you might need to use other indicators, such as weight circumference or an overall evaluation.

Your Ideal Weight

You need to achieve a point where you love your body. You will feel lighter but stronger. You will experience a feeling of being healthier. You will breathe better and have better skin and a better attitude. Your energy and sexual drive will increase. Finally, as you start loving your body more and more, you will feel happier.

Of course, identifying that set point can be tricky, but this is the most important aspect, as it will lead you to where you want to be. If you have been obese or really overweight for a long time, you might consider yourself in great physical shape after you lose some weight, but you are still far away from the healthy point. You need to make sure that, at a minimum, you are under the BMI and waist circumference limits recommended by health professionals.

If you have gained weight over a long period of time, and you might not know where you should be or where you could be, once you are sure you are below the IDF's recommendations based on your height and weight and you have mastered all the steps in this Program, you should continue using the knowledge you've gained. In fact, keep following this Program forever to see where it leads you.

Once your weight has stabilized and you are not losing or gaining weight, you have probably attained your perfect weight. But be realistic. If you have always been skinny and you want to go back to the figure you had in your twenties, you might keep fighting forever and never achieve your goal. We all need to accept that our bodies change with age, and it is difficult to be exactly the same as we were in our younger days.

You can't just sit back and accept adding weight every year as that will have no end. You need to check what your weight is right now, determine how different it is from maybe ten years ago, and find a point where you think you should be and where you feel comfortable, and where you can continue following this Program without too much trouble. You'll need to keep in control to maintain this approach and avoid deviating and gaining a little weight each month.

If you have only recently gained weight after having a bad time in your life, or following depression, divorce, pregnancy, or maybe having experienced too much fun in college or too much eating out after your first serious job, you probably still remember what your ideal weight is and where you want to be. You not only will be there after the thirty-two weeks, but you will learn the necessary steps to maintain your ideal weight forever and never allow yourself to stray that far away from where you want to be and should be.

Losing weight might be difficult if you have a low metabolic rate. There are several possible reasons for this, but none of them should make you throw in the towel on your weight loss goals. The 32 Mondays Weight Loss Program can truly help you overcome those difficulties; hormonal imbalance, aging, low thyroid function, chronic stress, insulin resistance, food addiction, depression, medication, excessive fat and yo-yo dieting are all addressed in the Program.

Where Should I Be?

By now, you can see why it is tricky to determine where you should be in terms of weight management. It can be personal, depending on how you want to see yourself, your age, genetics, nutrition knowledge, and other contributing factors.

In general, you need to at least accomplish three goals:

1. Your weight gives you a **BMI** below the overweight classification.

2. Your **waist circumference** is below the limit determined by the International Diabetes Federation to be considered at risk.

3. You feel comfortable with **how you see yourself**.

KEY POINTS

› Focus less on the scale and more on BMI and waist circumference.

› Focus on where you should be from a health point of view and how you see yourself.

› Determine and maintain your ideal weight.

PRINCIPLE 4
LEARNING TO TAKE CONTROL OF WHAT YOU EAT

There is no way to lose or maintain weight, to improve your health, and to gain energy and vitality if you can't take control of what you eat. And the only way to do that is to stop eating highly processed food. These are foods that have undergone significant transformation from the original natural ingredients. It is hard to determine what these products really contain and how they have been made or prepared. If you want to stop eating that way, there is no other choice but to start preparing your own food and take control of what you eat. To do so, you need to go back to the kitchen, start a food journal to know exactly what you are eating, and change your habits at the grocery store.

Bye-Bye to Fast, Highly Processed Food

We have become puppets. We no longer control what we feed our bodies. The food industry is doing it for us. They have brainstorming sessions to study the best way to connect specific flavors and textures to positive states of mind. Then, they manufacture products in such a way as to make us addicted to all those positive feelings and, finally, they develop great advertising campaigns to make us believe these foods are what we need! It's hard to resist a bag of potato chips when you're waiting somewhere and you find a vending machine, or a brownie in the afternoon when you are hungry and you walk by a coffee shop, or a big scoop of ice cream when you are finally ready to watch a movie on Friday night. The food industry also tries to make these foods as cheap as possible to make us think we are drawing huge pleasure while spending little money and experiencing great flavors. Soon we will be calling the process of eating unhealthy, highly processed food "a pleasant experience" or as the food industry calls it, "entertainment." And voilà! As David Kessler writes in *The End of Overeating*, "We have created the most powerful weapon against our bodies: ***fast, highly manufactured food.***"[3]

When you eat highly processed food from a fast food chain, you have no idea about all the unhealthy ingredients that have been included in that food and how it has been cooked.

When you eat food from a package, you are also eating those unhealthy ingredients, but at least you can recognize them—or most of them—by reading the labels. But chances are you don't have time to read the label, or if you do, you don't know how to interpret the effect on your body of 90 percent of the ingredients.

Let's take an example: monosodium glutamate (MSG). This is a flavor enhancer used widely in processed foods and restaurants. Its consumption in high quantities is associated with higher chances of being overweight. The reason is not clear. Maybe it is just that most of us eat more because of the enhanced taste, or maybe MSG impacts the way we metabolize fat. Either way, you should try to avoid its consumption as much as possible, but it is common in seasoning sauces, snack foods, salad dressings, and food in some restaurants.

≈

Processed foods are loaded with all sorts of artificial ingredients that serve as preservatives and flavor enhancers. And don't be fooled by the words *natural* or *all natural* on labels; those words can be misleading. Natural simply means that the food comes from nature and has not been artificially processed or modified. Natural does not necessarily mean healthy; the USDA definition of *natural* means the food **does** not contain artificial ingredients or preservatives and the ingredients are only minimally processed. However, they may contain antibiotics, growth hormones, and other similar chemicals.[4]

For example, a food might be loaded with "natural" salt or sugar. Let's compare labels from two different bottles of ranch dressing:

Ranch Salad Dressing

Ingredients

*Water, Soybean Oil, Sugar, Buttermilk Powder, contains 2% or less of each of the following: Salt, Distilled Vinegar, Modified Corn Starch, Phosphoric Acid, Xanthan Gum, Onion Powder, Garlic Powder, **Monosodium Glutamate**, Sorbic Acid and Calcium Disodium EDTA (used to protect quality), Polysorbate 60, Spices, Lemon Juice Concentrate, Propylene Glycol Alginate, Maltodextrin (Corn), Natural Flavor, Disodium Inosinate, Disodium Guanylate, Soy Lecithin.*

All Natural Ranch Dressing

Ingredients

Soybean Oil, Buttermilk, Distilled Vinegar, Egg Yolk, Salt, Sugar, Garlic*, Autolyzed Yeast Extract, Onion*, Spices, Xanthan Gum, Natural Flavors. *Dehydrated.

If you are concerned about paying more for healthier products, both examples cost the same per ounce, but the second one contains fewer artificial and unnecessary ingredients than the first one.

Don't let marketing trick you into thinking either of these is a healthy choice. Don't believe something is healthy unless you see it for real in the composition and food label. You *really* need to read the food label to be able to make the right decisions. Once you start reading food labels, you will start buying less of the bad options and more of the good ones. Even the same product—let's say two types of tomato sauce—can have different compositions. And often the taste of the healthier one is even better, though not necessarily more expensive.

As I said before, there is no way you can control your weight, figure, and health until you are able to control what you put into your body. And that, my friend, is not going to happen until you start taking control of what is used to prepare your foods.

Let's say, for example, you love cookies or muffins. As you will see later, most of the processed ones are made with nasty fats, including trans fats, which we'll discuss further in Step 6. That makes them not only high in calories, but also unhealthy. This doesn't mean you can't eat them anymore... you can always bake them at home to control the ingredients you use. If you don't like and/or don't have time to cook, you can use one of the high-quality organic mixes or eat an already-cooked organic cookie, which is usually lower in fats and trans fat-free. The same idea will apply for any other foods you absolutely love that are highly caloric and unhealthy. You can always find a healthier, less caloric choice. You simply need to look for it.

Another example is hydrogenated oils and fats. While the amount a product contains might be too low to be ranked as a trans fat in the Nutrition Facts, that nasty oil or fat is there.

Let's see a second example, this time about a pumpkin bread mix:

Pumpkin Bread Mix 1

Ingredients

Sugar, Enriched Bleached Flour (Wheat Flour, Malted Barley Flour, Niacin, Iron, Thiamin Mononitrate, Riboflavin, Folic Acid), Dried Pumpkin, Wheat Starch, **Partially Hydrogenated Soybean Oil**, *contains 2% or less of: Dextrose, Baking Powder (Baking Soda, Sodium Acid Pyrophosphate, Monocalcium Phosphate), Cinnamon, Nonfat Milk, Corn Starch, Spice,*

---

*Propylene Glycol Monoesters, Salt, Cellulose, Mono- and
Diglycerides, Colored with Yellow 5 and Red 40, Polysorbate 60,
Soy Lecithin, TBHQ and Citric Acid (Antioxidants).*

Pumpkin Bread Mix 2

Ingredients

*Unbleached Enriched Flour (Wheat Flour, Niacin, Reduced
Iron, Thiamin Mononitrate, Riboflavin, Folic Acid), Sugar,
Dried Pumpkin Flakes, Spices, Salt, Arabic Gum, Soybean Oil,
Leavening (Sodium Bicarbonate, Sodium Acid Pyrophosphate).*

Again, both bread mixes cost the same per ounce, but the second one does not contain partially hydrogenated soybean oil. Partially hydrogenated soybean oil is a trans fat, but the amount included per serving size is low enough to avoid having to list it.

The second mix only has the ingredients necessary to make a good pumpkin bread, avoiding unnecessary colors, as well as mono- and diglycerides, among others.

There are many other examples, like a long list of unrecognizable sugars that are included in many products that add to the amount of sugar we consume on a daily basis. You will find a list of those sugars in Appendix D.

If you want to win the battle against the food manufacturing industry, you may have to re-educate your taste buds to love other textures, flavors, and senses. One example of succeeding in this is moving to whole grain ingredients or new products. By learning how to nourish your body with adequate foodstuffs, you will be in control of the battle.

Processed food is so refined and so easy to eat that we consume thousands of calories without even realizing it. Think about the difference between an apple and applesauce. How long does it take to eat one and the other? What about apple juice? And we are talking here about healthy stuff! But what about the extra sugar in sauces, added to make them even more desirable and easier to eat? And what of all the precooked and ready-to-eat meals that contain added fat, sugar, and salt to make them more visually appealing, tasty, and addictive?

Palatability

If you'd like to read more about how the food industry is manipulating the way you eat, read *The End of Overeating*. In it, Kessler explains how the food industry has investigated ways to make food more palatable, meaning not just that it has an agreeable taste, but that it stimulates our appetite, making us not only eat more, but pursue that taste. According to Kessler, the most palatable food contains a high combination of sugar, fat, and salt. The food industry searches for the perfect combination to make food not just palatable, but what Kessler calls "hyper-palatable." They make us desire that food and come back again and again in pursuit of not only that taste, but the whole experience for all our senses. Sounds manipulative, doesn't it? Well, it is, and it also makes us use a specific food as a reward, or even obsess about that food to the point of getting addicted to it.

I know this sounds scary, but it doesn't mean you can't break the trap of manipulation by the food industry. I can assure you that once you stop eating that food and get used to healthier options, you won't miss your old habits at all. In fact, you will begin craving the good stuff, and your new, healthy body will be addicted to it. But there is no way this can happen if you don't know specifically what your food contains. To do so, you need to go back to the kitchen and the grocery store to gain control of what you eat most of the time.

Back to the Kitchen

If you want to manage your weight, your figure, your health, and your state of mind by taking control of what you feed your body, you need to go back to the kitchen. That doesn't mean you have to spend thousands of hours organizing meals, developing skills worthy of a chef, or spending lots of money on kitchen utensils and sophisticated meals. Healthy eating does not require a natural ability to cook. What you need is a high dose of motivation to change your habits and become incredibly efficient at the grocery store and in your kitchen. You will learn how in the next two chapters.

Choose the Right Foods

Now that you know how the manufacturing industry is manipulating the way you eat, you need to learn to choose the right foods. Instead of yielding to the attraction of specific foods, think first about what they contain. Ask yourself:

> › How will my body react to them?

> › How will I feel after a short period of time?

> › Will these foods satiate me, or will they make me feel hungrier?

Do not just go and eat. Think first, and try to make the right choice. You will learn more about those choices in the following chapters. For example, if you let your body run low of sugar, you are going to feel irritable and anxious, which will lead you to make poor food choices. However, if you prepare in advance and don't let your sugar levels drop by having a healthy and fulfilling snack at the right time, you will not face those problems. You will learn a lot more about this with the 32 Mondays Weight Management Program.

KEY POINTS

> › Avoid highly processed food.

> › Read labels.

> › Learn how the food industry is manipulating you.

> › Choose your food wisely.

PRINCIPLE 5
MASTERING GROCERY SHOPPING

Once you know about the aspects we covered in Principles 1 through 4, you have to work on your behavior at the grocery store. Grocery stores are better called "festival stores." All of your senses are stimulated when you arrive there. Everything is well presented, colorful, and looks delicious. As you walk down the aisles, the aroma of freshly baked bread, the scent of fruit, and the colorful packaging of other food appeal to your senses. As you start savoring all those products, you feel like you are starving and are ready to buy and eat everything. In ways similar to the food manufacturing industry, grocery store chains know exactly how to convince you to buy much more than you would ever need.

Supermarket layouts have been designed to make it difficult to find basic products and instead make you wander around the aisles so you see products that you might desire and end up buying. This is why you'll see changes to the organization of the supermarket from time to time.

For your long-term health, you must learn which products to buy, in which store you'll find those, and exactly where they are located in the store. This is not a quick or easy process, but once you have mastered it, your grocery shopping will be tremendously simplified. When you know the layout of your preferred supermarkets, you can focus on what you need and avoid the "enemy" aisles full of unnecessary stuff.

Two Rules for Successful Grocery Shopping

The first rule of healthy eating is to never, ever go to the grocery store when you are hungry. You cannot think rationally when you're hungry. You can only focus on what you can do to fulfill a basic need: nourishment. How are you going to focus on buying healthy foods when your brain is obsessed about getting some direct sugar to make it work? Your brain is an organ that constantly needs a quick and easy-to-use form of energy—sugar—so it will send the hormonal team to make you desire, crave, buy, and eat basic and simple energy: *sugar*! Your subconscious will send you right to the chocolate doughnuts aisle to make you buy those high-sugar, high-fat bombs.

The best time to shop for your groceries is after a nourishing meal.

I am usually strict with my grocery shopping list, but whenever I go to the grocery store feeling hungry, I always end up buying some unhealthy products for myself and my kids.

The second rule when going to the grocery store is to avoid going with your kids. They'll distract you from the main objectives: to read food labels, locate good deals, and buy only what's necessary. Children also have the ability to make you buy sugary food, candy, bakery items, and other products that you wouldn't have bought if you were on your own. If you have to take them with you, use the opportunity to practice what you have learned and teach them about healthy eating.

How to Plan a Successful Grocery Shopping Trip

The tips for success at the grocery store are organization and some initial investment in time. Start right by changing your view of your grocery store. Learn where to buy your products and where to find them in your preferred stores. You will need to have all this information in just five weeks once you start the 32 Mondays Weight Management Program.

First, you have to spend some time at each store to learn what products you'll purchase from each one, paying attention to their quality and price. Examples of products you will search for and compare include organic fruit, vegetables, and milk, ready-to-microwave vegetables, organic meat and chicken, whole-grain bread and cereals, and wild fish. You need to know in exactly which aisle these products are located. You also need to plan on a specific route to follow in each store. Every time you go to that store, you will need to follow a predetermined and specific route to avoid missing any of the products you buy there so you don't have to come back. More important, when you see your preferred products on sale, you'll want to stock up if possible.

You might end up shopping in several different stores. However, once you know what to buy in each one and where the products are located, the shopping routine will become easier and quicker than you expect. If you follow the route in each one with no deviation, you should be able to get your groceries in the same amount of time as you invested shopping haphazardly in just one store. Additionally, if you keep focused on the route, you will avoid being tempted to buy all the things you don't really need, which will save you money and unhealthy food. Remember the doughnuts we were talking about before?

You may need a few "field trips" to your preferred supermarkets to learn about each specific store and to decide where to buy each product. Not every store or chain has the same products. They sometimes have non-competition agreements on certain products, and even suppliers determine to whom they distribute different products. For example, I love an organic brand that has ham, turkey, prosciutto, and similar products. My family loves the ham. There are two chain stores very close to each other that carry that brand. One has the ham and the other carries the turkey. So if I want both, I'll have to make a trip to each store. A pain? Yes, but that is how it is, and that is why you need to become efficient at the grocery store to save as much time as possible.

If you can't stay away from buying non-appropriate products while at the grocery store, always carry a shopping list, or shop online.

Another good recommendation for healthy food is to shop at a farmer's market. Check out *http://apps.ams.usda.gov/farmersmarkets* to see what is available in your area.

Meal Planning

Plan your meals according to product availability. Let's say that organic chicken and mushrooms are on sale. Buy extra. Cook a large amount of chicken with mushrooms and freeze the leftovers to be eaten in two weeks' time. I recommend using transparent containers to see and keep track of what's in your refrigerator and freezer.

Extra Stock

Some of the healthier products are more expensive than conventional ones and cheap brands. Other products, contrary to what people think, are not. For most food, it is worth paying the extra cost to get the benefits. When products you like are on sale or at reduced prices, I suggest you buy extra. If they are perishable and need to be used soon, think about meals you can prepare with them right then, and stock the rest for a few days until you can use them or freeze them. Remember, the life of a product is extended once you cook it, and you can freeze the leftovers for later in the week. If you learn how to shop sales and stock up or use products before they exceed their expiration date, you can save much more money than you would ever think you could, and compensate for some of the extra cost of the healthier food.

Managing the extra stock you buy is simply a matter of organization: make room for nonperishable items in your cabinets. Clean out your refrigerator and remove things that don't really need to be refrigerated. Organize the refrigerator and freezer to make room for your fresh products and cooked meals.

In **Appendix E** you will find a list of products to locate in your preferred supermarkets. Make your grocery store list using the template, or use this suggested list:

> › **Essentials** you always buy—milk, fruit, vegetables, ham, cheese, yogurt, bread, fish, chicken

> › **Weekly ingredients**—beef, mushrooms, half and half, chicken thighs

> › **Special offers** for the week—organic blueberries or strawberries,

organic chicken broth, tomato juice, olive oil, special fish, or meat to freeze

› **Staples**—soap, napkins, pasta, rice, toilet paper, spices

Keep your lists on your computer so you can modify them quickly each week to take advantage of your meal planning and the specials at your favorite grocery stores. Over time, you will learn to have everything in your mind and you won't need a list to remind you what to buy and which specials to check every time.

KEY POINTS

› Never go to the grocery store when hungry.

› Try to avoid bringing the kids to the supermarket.

› Make a list and follow it or buy online if you can't avoid buying extras.

› Buy at your local farmer's market.

› Learn where your basic products are located in each store.

› Plan your meals according to product availability.

› Buy extra stock when on sale.

› Organize your kitchen to allow for extra stock.

PRINCIPLE 6
NAVIGATING THE KITCHEN

You already know that to succeed in your weight, figure, and health management, you need to take control of what you eat. You have learned how to manage shopping for your food. Now it is time to learn what to do with it.

If you don't cook, this is the right time to start. I know it sounds scary, and I know you think you will never be able to survive the kitchen. But listen, you don't have to be a renowned chef to learn to prepare enough meals to move to a healthy lifestyle and start to be in control of your weight. If cooking is not your thing and you really can't do it, just learn which veggies are microwavable, how to fix a salad, and learn to cook a simple egg and how to sauté or stir-fry meat or fish. Those simple and basic cooking skills will lead you though the program until you are interested in learning more about cooking.

I am aware that cooking even the simplest recipe can take a crazy amount of time. You have to prepare the ingredients, cook them, serve them, and clean up the mess. If you are like 99 percent of us, you have more commitments and obligations than free time. Some of you love to cook but only have time to do so during the weekends. Others don't even like cooking but do it because they already recognize the importance of home-cooked meals. The rest have never cooked or don't like cooking. But now that you are aware of the importance of what you eat, it's time to prepare your own meals.

Organize Your Cooking Time

The first step to succeed in cooking your meals is to organize your cooking time. No matter what you cook or your preparation method, it won't be useful if you don't find the time and energy to cook.

The good news is that if you can manage to find one hour a day to cook, you are fine. That is all you need, including preparation, cooking, and clean up. But you need to be focused during that time. Give it the same importance in terms of concentration as you would give a task at work, or the importance you recommend your children give to homework.

If you cannot manage one hour a day, you need to find some additional time on a specific day or over the weekend to cook meals for the rest of the week. Let's say on Wednesdays, you have two hours to cook dinner. Don't spend them preparing a super-fancy dinner and then eat something from a box the rest of the week. Use the extra time you have available to prepare meals for the other days of the week.

Are you having a barbecue over the weekend? Cook some extra sausages and zucchini to have ready for one lunch the next week, and some chicken drumsticks and corn to have for one dinner. Barbecue adds different flavors, which will give you the opportunity to eat a different meal during the week when you don't have time for a barbecue. Maybe during the week you can make a chicken soup with vegetables and zucchini with the extra stock you bought because there was a great deal in the organic section. But because the flavor of the stir-fry or soup is very different than the barbecue you had over the weekend, you won't get bored with chicken and zucchini.

Do you see how this works? It is basically a matter of being smart in the kitchen and creating additional opportunities for extra lunches or dinners, or at least having enough leftovers to cover a meal when you don't have time to cook. So always try to cook extra food to have ready in the refrigerator or the freezer to use when you don't have time to cook, you are exhausted, or in any other special or emergency situation.

Ready-to-use vegetables or even healthy precooked meals are also a big ally. You can have vegetables in the fridge or freezer, and you will always have some greens available and ready to use. If you are smart at reading labels, you can find healthy soups and even precooked meats that can be stored in the fridge or even in the pantry and are ready to use. Look at the ingredients and avoid sugars, hydrogenated fats, canola oil when possible, and check that they don't contain too much salt. Usually, organic foods are the best choice when eating prepared foods. They are not packed with preservatives and ugly color additives and generally do not use genetically modified ingredients.

In Step 4 of the 32 Mondays Weight Management Program, you will find the details about how many meals per day you should be having and how to organize them. As you will learn (and contrary to what many people are used to), I recommend making lunch your main meal and then having a frugal dinner. By lunchtime you still have a long way to go in your day, so you need energy. By dinnertime, you are close to bedtime, so your energy requirements are much lower. Also, while you are sleeping a weight management-friendly hormone team works to help you manage your weight, and that team works *much* better when there is little energy available and the hunger hormone ghrelin has been vanquished. You'll learn more about this in Principle 9.

And yes, both lunch and dinner should always be as close to homemade as possible—no snack-based meals or highly processed foods.

Cooking for the Family

Chances are, if your eating habits aren't what they should be and have resulted in poor health and extra weight, your family probably suffers from the same problems. If you think you need to change your life and eat better, you would probably like your loved ones to do the same.

If you have family to cook for, there is no way you are going to be able to manage your time if you need to cook two different meals a day for you and two more for the rest of the family. That makes four meals each day! Your family also deserves a healthy future and a well-managed weight, so move them all to your new way of eating and prepare the same meals for all of you. It might take them some time to get used to, but if you stay determined, they will get used to it, and by teaching them how to eat, you'll be giving them a gift for the rest of their lives. When your needs are different from the rest of the family's because your goal is weight loss, or if you are less active, your percentage of greens and protein should be greater than the rest of your family's, and you should eat fewer carbohydrates. If their energy needs are still not met with the meals you are preparing, add additional healthy calories to their meal with some extra nuts, some dark chocolate, a yogurt, or a healthy cookie.

Lunch: Your Main Meal of the Day

As I wrote above, lunch should be a much more substantial meal than dinner. It needs to include some carbohydrates for energy, protein for long-term maintenance, healthy fats to help you feel full, and vegetables and fruits for vitamins and minerals. (We'll discuss the importance of this composition for meals in Step 4.) Carbohydrates include bread, pasta, rice, legumes, and cereals. Protein includes meat, fish, chicken, ham, salami, cheese, tofu (soya), beans, and nuts.

The basic secret to cooking creatively for yourself and your family is to master seven easy meals, one for each day of the week. You'll find examples of a menu plan for a week with the recipes at the end of the book, or you can use your own favorites. You can also substitute a meal replacement or protein shake for one of your meals each day. My favorite ones are from Arbonne (check *www.arantxamateo.arbonne.com*). You can get the powder to prepare the shakes or have the ready-to-drink ones for more convenience.

If you eat lunch at the office, at school, or anywhere away from home, prepare meals that are easy to eat (no chicken drumsticks, for example) and not too smelly (fish, cauliflower, Indian spices). You have to learn to make these meals so well that you can almost prepare them with your eyes closed. If you or someone in your family has ever played an instrument, you'll know that practice makes perfect. I believe that is true for most daily activities: driving, ice skating, dancing, climbing, cycling on two wheels—and now cooking. Once you have mastered your seven meals to cover the week, you can start experimenting with them.

For example, let's say you have mastered chicken with mushrooms. Your next step is change things a bit to create a new version: one week you can exchange the mushrooms for other vegetables; another week you can change the type of chicken (thighs instead of breasts); and every week you can serve it with a different carbohydrate like brown rice, whole-wheat pasta, quinoa, or whole-grain couscous. Combinations of the three variables (chicken, vegetables, and carbohydrates) gives you an important variety of dishes during the week so you don't have to repeat them often.

Look at the number of combinations you can get with only a few ingredients:

	Chicken	Beef	Ground Beef/ Chicken
Whole Wheat Pasta	1	2	3
Brown Rice	4	5	6
Whole Couscous	7	8	9
Quinoa	10	11	12

And if with each variable you introduce a different vegetable, for example, you add four new combinations for meals using that protein. Be creative and add different sauces and spices to add flavors to your recipe.

Let's face it: having to cook every single meal for yourself or for the whole family can get tiring and boring. Use your creativity and imagination to create your own unique recipes and have fun during the process to keep your meals healthy and varied.

Some recipes will not allow for too many variations. You should keep those to use every other week or every two weeks. You'll find an example of a weekly meal plan in Appendix F.

Another tip to make meals more appealing is to add something interesting to the menu. Let's say that fish is not your or your family's favorite food. Well, reserve some treats for the day you cook fish, like ice cream, cake, a piece of chocolate, some lemonade, or a candy. Then the day you have rich macaroni with meat, eat only fruit as a dessert.

Dinner Meals

You will be eating a light, home-cooked meal for dinner, which includes vegetables and some light protein (egg, tofu, fish, cheese, etc.), with some fruit or dairy product like yogurt or kefir (a fermented dairy product similar to yogurt but more liquid and less acidic). Here again you can play with the ingredient combinations, including fruits and desserts. For example, one week you can make scrambled eggs and mushrooms and another week a mushroom omelet. Same ingredients, different presentation. After a light dinner, and if you haven't had your treat during the day, you can have a small treat (a square of dark chocolate, a small homemade cookie, a small scoop of ice cream, five candied nuts, or five to ten potato chips if that's your preference).

KEY POINTS

› Prepare some basic meals to succeed in your weight management objective.

› Organization is the key to successful home cooking.

› Find one hour a day for cooking or some extra time during the week or over the weekend to prepare meals for the entire week.

› Lunch should be your main meal of the day.

› Prepare extra food and store for emergencies.

› Cook the same food for the whole family.

› Start by mastering seven meals and combine ingredients to create more varieties.

› If you eat well during the day, have a treat, but don't eat all high-calorie foods in the same meal.

PRINCIPLE 7
PHYSICAL AND PSYCHOLOGICAL FOOD ADDICTIONS

There are many books and opinions about food addiction and weight management—almost as many as there are different approaches to weight management and diets, and certainly enough to confuse you.

Some diet book authors argue that it is only your ability to refrain from eating that counts. For others, brain mechanisms (some controllable, some not) are the most important cause for being overweight. The truth probably lies neither at one end nor the other, but somewhere in the middle: your own self-control and your subconscious mind determine what, when, and how much you eat.

There is a certain pattern behind your reaction to foods that you know you shouldn't be eating. It feels like a force pushing you toward those "bad" foods. It feels like an addiction. Earlier we discussed how the food manufacturing industry manipulates food to exercise control over your will. In more precise terms, the food industry aims to manipulate you so you'll consume more and more of their products. These highly modified foods are not good for you, especially if your objective is to gain control over your weight and become healthier. The truth is that some of those products really have some addictive power over you. Learning about this addictive power will help you manage it.

There are two types of addiction: physical and psychological. Both of these mechanisms are in play when we talk about eating behavior.

Physical Food Addiction

Physical addiction occurs when your body becomes used to a certain substance. After some time, it becomes difficult to function properly without it. This type of addiction is difficult to manage because the moment you don't take those substances, there is a withdrawal effect that makes you feel miserable physically. The only way to restore your body to a normal function is to remove the addictive substance so the body learns how to function without that substance. The good news about physical food addiction is that once you overcome the withdrawal process, you will not feel more negative effects— unless you are again exposed to the same substance. This new exposure will trigger the addiction once more, and you will need to go through the same withdrawal process.

Some people show a high addiction to certain foods, especially those that combine fat, sugar, and salt, like cookies, doughnuts, muffins, crackers, and some kinds of potato chips. Unlike other types of physical addictions, breaking the physical addiction to these foods is relatively easy.

When you eat a specific addictive food, there is a glucose peak and consequently a high insulin response. When glucose is suddenly removed by insulin, there is a big drop in glucose levels. This is followed by a craving effect—you search for more of the addictive food. If you can resist this specific craving, the physical addiction of this cycle will be over soon. Fortunately, when you change your eating and exercising habits while following the 32 Mondays Weight Management Program, you will have other alternatives, and you will start to crave healthy foods and a healthy lifestyle that will help you break those addictive cycles. You'll win the battle over the physical addiction and its related hormones by understanding them.

Psychological Food Addiction

Psychological addiction is much more complex than the physical addiction. The difficulty is not only the complexity of our minds but also the lack of knowledge about most of the mechanisms that take place in our minds. We are all different, so we respond differently to external stimuli. For some of us, food can have a palliative effect when we are depressed or in trouble. Other people won't be able to eat anything in those same situations.

Many of us tend to think that food helps us when we feel down by providing us with some pleasure. Food is also associated to a pleasant night out, an afternoon movie, a happy breakfast, or any such merry occasion. The problem arises when you associate food with those feelings. Food cannot give you a pleasant night out unless you have a good partner or friend to enjoy the night, or a good movie, or music, or a good restaurant. If you are not happy with what you have, food is not going to add any more happiness.

A chocolate bar will give you instant pleasure while you are eating it, but that happiness will turn to smoke as soon as the bar is finished. With physical addiction, the moment you don't feed the addictive substance to your body, you can physically feel the withdrawal experience and become aware of what is going on. With psychological addiction, you don't really feel anything but the instant pleasure of it, so you think you are happy or unhappy because of that. Food can end up being a real obsession.

> *Happiness comes from the inside, not from whatever enters your mouth.*

Recognize and accept that food will not give you anything you don't have. If you are happy with your life, a good meal will add pleasure to it. If you feel miserable, you will feel the same way after you eat a burger, lasagna, a candy bar, a doughnut, or a bag of chips. Once you have truly accepted this reality, you will stop having so many cravings for unhealthy food.

Social Pressure

Social pressure is one of the main causes of psychological addiction. Society teaches us to constantly seek rewards: "I want it and I want it now!" We seek success and reward for everything we do: jobs and careers (be successful, earn more money); friendships (be accepted); relationships (be loved); school (get good grades); sports (be an achiever); and physical image (be slim). At the same time, our society is becoming more demanding, more competitive, and more exacting. It is more difficult to feel successful than ever before; to be rewarded for our efforts and sacrifices is increasingly rare. While this ever-increasing pressure has developed, the food industry has found the exact recipe to fill that void. **We can now feel rewarded when we eat certain foods because they've been scientifically developed for enhanced taste and palatability.**

> *Food marketers continuously bombard us with messages like, "Eat this and you will feel great, empowered, energized," and "You deserve it for all your efforts, your tensions, your pressure! You deserve your reward." Not that long ago, food was simply a way to get nourished and energized. Later we learned how food could provide us with pleasure. Today we have learned how to use food as a reward to the point of obsession about some foods and even psychological addiction. We need to learn that food can be more or less tasteful or pleasurable, but it can never substitute for anything or fill voids in your life. Fight for the real thing— career, friends, success, or real love—and leave food just to celebrate what you have accomplished!*

Food addiction reminds me a lot of nicotine addiction. If you think you have a food addiction or even a nicotine problem, I urge you to read one of my favorite books about addiction: Allen Carr's *Easy Way to Stop Smoking.*

Bad Habits

As if social pressure wasn't bad enough, now you have your own bad habits: skipping breakfast, the "fridge attack" as soon as you get home, a bag of chips and a Coke while watching TV, the super-mega-buttered popcorn and a huge box of candy at the movie theater, nachos with mega-fatty cheese dip when having a beer with friends, chocolate cookies while having an afternoon coffee… the list can get really long. The worst part is that you eat all of these terribly unhealthy foods without even experiencing a tiny little sense of hunger. Sometimes, you don't even realize you are eating! These foods are just adding calories. Worse, they are adding inches to your waist.

Another bad habit is eating until you're stuffed. Think about how slow and heavy you feel when you eat that way and think about how long it takes you to get back to "normal" functioning. Adopt the new habit of leaving the table when you are just satisfied.

Make a list of your bad habits and stick it on the door of your refrigerator. Put additional copies of the list on your office desk, on your sofa, and any other place you spend time, and liberate yourself from those terrifying bad habits!

When you follow the 32 Mondays Weight Management Program, you will end your bad habits and develop good ones. When following each step and allowing the required time to settle into the new routine and recommendations, you will change your subconscious habits without even realizing you're doing so.

BEING HUNGRY VERSUS FEELING LIKE EATING

One of the most common bad habits many of us have is eating when we aren't really hungry. Physical hunger, actual hunger, comes gradually. It starts with a growling stomach that grows until you start to feel physically ill. A headache and tiredness start if you don't eat something. When you are hungry, you become flexible about your food options, and you can't wait to be fed. Once you are full, you feel better and you stop eating. Finally, you are free of guilt.

On the other hand, "I feel like eating something" comes suddenly as an unstoppable desire to eat something specific, often one of the addictive foods: something sweet, salty, and fatty. You can't wait. You have to eat it *right now*, and you keep eating and eating until you are *really* full. You feel guilty soon after.

See the difference? Learn to anticipate which feeling you are experiencing and how to proceed depending on the available options: the right snack or a smart delay in your immediate desire for satisfaction. You will learn to do this in Step 4 when you learn how to organize your meals.

KEY POINTS

> Addiction to food can be physical and/or psychological. Physical addiction can be overcome by refusing to buy into manipulation by the food industry and instead eating healthy foods.

> Psychological addictions, including social pressure, are more difficult to fight. You need to recognize them and make an effort to change the pattern.

> Food cannot be a substitute for values, experiences, and feelings that are important, including friendship and love. Don't use food as a proxy for good experiences.

> Bad habits can be changed into good ones if you learn to recognize them.

> Learn the difference between being hungry and feeling like eating something.

PRINCIPLE 8
ALL ABOUT INSULIN

Insulin is so important that it needs a chapter by itself. You really need to learn and understand about insulin and how it works so you can manage your weight. It is one of the principal components of this weight management plan. We will refer to this chapter in several of the steps.

What Is Insulin?

Insulin is the hormone responsible for removing glucose, the simplest form of carbohydrate (simply stated: sugars), from your bloodstream and carrying it to the cells in your body. Glucose must be removed from the bloodstream for two reasons: first, you need its energy to feed your cells and organs, and second, high quantities of glucose in your bloodstream are toxic for your body.

How Insulin Works

The pancreas, one of your internal organs, is responsible for generating insulin in the beta cells. The quantity it generates depends on the quantity of glucose in the bloodstream at a specific moment. Several indicators—all related to the amount and composition of food eaten, how much fat and muscle you have in your body, and whether you have just exercised, among other things—will signal the amount of insulin the pancreas needs to produce. Once insulin is released into the bloodstream, it sticks to glucose and helps it travel into the cells of different organs depending on specific energy needs.

Once your immediate energy needs are covered, the excess glucose is stored as glycogen in the liver and, if there is still any left, as body fat. Put simply, if you have more glucose than needed, the body will store it as fat.

You will see later how it is important that you maintain steady glucose and insulin levels; this is the way the body works best.

How Your Body Balances Energy

After each meal, food is digested in the intestines, with each type of energy— simple sugars, proteins, carbohydrates, and fats—absorbed at a different pace in the intestine.

Simple carbohydrates—like table sugar and candies—are absorbed from the intestine into the bloodstream quickly as simple glucose.

More complex carbohydrates—such as wheat and rice—take longer because they need to be modified into simpler sugars (glucose) first.

Very complex carbohydrates—including whole grains and some vegetables—not only take more time to digest, but part of those sugars may not be absorbed at all because they are retained between the fiber that makes up whole grains and vegetables. Fiber is not absorbed.

Fats break into simple forms (fatty acids) and are absorbed like that. **Proteins** are transformed into amino acids before being absorbed. **Both protein and fat slow the absorption of glucose into the bloodstream.**

Glucose moves rapidly to the bloodstream, where it is removed by insulin to feed the main glucose-consuming organ, your brain, and then the other organs. When there is more glucose than needed, insulin removes the excess and brings it to the liver where it is transformed temporarily into glycogen until needed. If it is not needed because you have fulfilled your requirements with basic glucose, or the liver has reached its capacity to store more quantity, glycogen is transformed into triglycerides—a type of fat—and it is deposited as fatty tissue in different parts of the body.

When glucose runs too low to be able to fulfill the requirements of different organs, another important hormone, **glucagon** (which is secreted by the pancreas's alpha cells) transforms glycogen into glucose to be directly used. If there is still not enough glucose, it will go to the fat deposits to transform fat into triglycerides and then into glucose.

Your organs—especially your brain, which can't use any other source of energy—always use sugars (glucose) as a primary source of energy. **Fats will only be used once sugars and glycogen have been consumed.** This is especially true with your muscles when exercising. Amino acids from proteins are building blocks for your body—especially for your muscles—and are only used as a source of energy as a last resource, which is basically when you are fasting.

That's why when planning your exercise routine it is recommended you first do anaerobic exercise (weight lifting or similar exercise) to consume all the glucose and glycogen easily available and then go for an aerobic exercise (running or something similar). In this way, the body accesses fat deposits as a source of energy during aerobic exercise (running), once glucose and glycogen are all consumed during the anaerobic exercise (weight lifting). See Step 11 for more information.

The most important point here is to exercise long enough to consume glucose and glycogen (best accomplished by anaerobic exercise), and to keep exercising when they are no longer available so the body must burn stored fat for energy. Medium-intensity aerobic exercise favors fat burning.

By the way, for each gram of glycogen the body stores, it stores 3 grams of water, too. This is one of the reasons you lose weight so quickly when you follow one of the multiple diets that restrict carbohydrates: you basically lose all the water attached to glycogen. When no glucose is available because there are no carbohydrates in the diet, your body is forced to burn all the glycogen available, and therefore the water attached to the glycogen is lost. You will recover that water again as soon as you eat carbohydrates again and restore your glycogen deposits.

Pancreas Burnout and Excess Fat Storage

If you constantly eat foods with a high proportion of simple sugars (glucose, fructose) or simple carbohydrates (white bread, rice, and pasta), you overload the pancreas, and it must constantly secrete insulin. This affects your weight metabolism and ends up breaking the equilibrium, making you gain weight. After years of mistreating your pancreas, its activity will decrease in the long term, and it will lose its ability to generate insulin and regulate glucose in the bloodstream. When that happens, you can end up pre-diabetic or diabetic. Additionally, your body loses its ability to manage the excess energy (in terms of food transformed into glucose), and it becomes less efficient at burning the excess energy, instead storing it as fat.

Therefore, **it is extremely important that you always maintain low sugar levels**, but high enough to provide enough energy to go through your normal daily life. You will learn how to do so in practice in several of the steps of 32 Mondays Weight Management Program.

Here is an association I find useful when I need to remember the effects of highly glycemic food in an empty stomach, using candy as a stand-in for glucose, children's behavior as a stand-in for insulin, and parents as a stand-in for the pancreas.

You go to a kids' party. They have been playing and running the whole afternoon. They are starving. No food has been served yet. It is piñata time! The piñata is full of candy (glucose). The kids (insulin) break the piñata and start to take as much candy as possible. The parents (pancreas) keep trying to control the kids' behavior (insulin), but there is so much candy and so many kids going crazy for the candy that everybody loses control. The parents are exhausted and can't manage their kids anymore, and they finally decide to just give up and let them do whatever they want. The kids go crazy eating eat candy and become hyperactive (insulin resistance, diabetes type II) as a consequence of all the candy (glucose) ingested.

Glycemic Index

Glycemic index (GI) is a measure of the effect of a specific carbohydrate in blood glucose. Understanding this concept will help you maintain healthy blood sugar levels, which makes a huge difference for both weight loss and weight maintenance.

Foods with a low GI make blood glucose rise gently and therefore do not activate a high insulin response. Examples of carbohydrates with low GI are vegetables and whole grains. Foods with high amounts of fiber also have lower GI. Although they can be more or less caloric, the insulin response is under control, and so are the cravings for more sugar.

On the other hand, carbohydrates with high GI (direct sugars, white grains, potatoes) cause a high increase in glucose, with the subsequent high-insulin response. Once the high levels of insulin enter the bloodstream and glucose levels drop, you experience an immediate craving for sugar and an increase in appetite. Avoid high GI carbohydrates, or at least make sure that whenever you eat them, you accompany them with protein and fat in the same meal to reduce the glucose spike.

GI foods are classified as follows:

› **GI> 70 High**

› **69 > GI > 56 Medium**

› **GI < 55 Low**

Here are a few **examples** of food in each category:

› **High**: white bread, white rice, potato, rice milk, rice crackers, watermelon

› **Medium**: raisins, cantaloupe, brown rice, sweet potato, ice cream, orange juice

› **Low**: whole-grain bread, beans, yogurt, wheat pasta, all nuts, most fruits and vegetables

An interesting point to consider is how different types of breads and rice fall into different classifications. The more fiber (especially soluble fiber) a food contains—examples include grain bread, brown rice, and beans—the lower the GI. While oranges are considered low in GI, orange juice falls in the medium category because the fiber is removed when juicing.

Glycemic Load

The glycemic load (GL) of food is also a number that estimates how much the food will raise your blood glucose level. Unlike glycemic index, glycemic load considers how much carbohydrate is in the food, how much each gram of carbohydrate in the food raises blood glucose levels, and the portion size when you eat that food. Glycemic load is based on the GI, and it is defined as the grams of available carbohydrate in the food times the food's GI divided by 100.

For instance, watermelon has a high GI (73), but carbohydrates make up only 5 percent of a typical serving, so the glycemic effect of eating it (and therefore its GL) is low (3.6). Bread (white and whole wheat) has a similar behavior in terms of GI and GL.

On the other side, pasta has a low GI (52), but because you tend to eat a lot in a serving and it has a high content of carbohydrate, its GL is high (23) for a serving size of one cup.

This is the reason you should consider not only the GI value of a food, but also its GL value.

Whereas glycemic index is defined for each type of food, glycemic load can be calculated for any size serving of a food, an entire meal, or an entire day's meals because it depends on how many carbohydrates are consumed.

GL foods are classified as follows:

› **GL> 20 High**

› **19 > GL > 11 Medium**

› **GL < 10 Low**

Here are a few **examples** of food in each category:

› **High:** pasta, couscous, white rice, potato, corn flakes

› **Medium:** banana, sweet potato, wild rice, orange juice

› **Low:** beans, nuts, most fresh fruits and vegetables

For more detailed information, visit *www.glycemicindex.com* and *www. mendosa.com.*

Try keeping a list with the GI and GL values of the foods you eat most until you have learned about them.

While glycemic index and glycemic load are good reference values to determine the glucose impact (and therefore the insulin response) a food creates in your body, they can't be considered in isolation. While learning how to manage your weight appropriately, you should consider all the other aspects and conditions explained and covered in the 32 Mondays Weight Management Program.

Care and Treatment of Your Pancreas

Your pancreas plays an important role in your weight management story by providing the necessary insulin to balance glucose levels, especially its peaks. You need to treat this organ well and consider it to maintain optimum health.

If you want to be your pancreas's friend, this is how to help it:

1. **Learn about the glycemic index (GI) and glycemic load (GL) of food and limit the amount of high-glycemic food you ingest.** If your pancreas is always working too hard, it will tire and become less effective.

2. **Give your pancreas a rest.** It needs at least three to four hours to rest between shifts, which means three to four hours between each meal.

3. **Never have high-glycemic foods by themselves.** When you eat glucose alone, it pushes the pancreas to generate as much insulin as possible to remove the glucose as soon as possible. Those candies you eat to alleviate your hunger not only hit your pancreas hard, but they also

have the opposite effect and don't alleviate hunger, as you will see later. Always eat high-glycemic foods like sugar, chocolate, sugary or alcoholic drinks, pasta, rice, and fruit, with protein and fat, and, when possible, at the end of a meal. If there is something else in your stomach, especially some protein or fat, insulin won't be wandering around by itself trying to reduce the amount of glucose in your bloodstream.

4. **Exercise before eating.** You will deplete your glycogen reserves during exercise instead of storing the energy contained in the food ingested as fat. Then when you do eat, the glucose levels in your blood will be under control because the glucose will be immediately transformed into glycogen in the liver to be used later when needed.

Health Effects of Poor Insulin Management

Weight gain and obesity are the most common consequences of poor insulin management. When you continue pushing beta cells from the pancreas to produce insulin, insulin resistance can occur, which could result in prediabetes and type II diabetes.

Insulin resistance develops after a disruption in the insulin-glucose equilibrium takes place. It could be caused by sickness or an external factor, but in most cases, it is due to a systematic excess of glucose consumption and out-of-control insulin production, and also as a consequence of fat accumulation in your abdomen because of bad eating habits or a genetic predisposition. Cells that are sensitive to insulin tire of working all the time and end up not giving an adequate response when insulin is present; they become insulin resistant. As a result, they can't remove glucose from the bloodstream, and you suffer an increase in blood glucose. The pancreas detects it and responds by producing a still-higher amount of insulin until a response is generated, and glucose is removed.

In an insulin-resistant or prediabetes situation, glucose levels remain high until they drop in a rapid fall. This happens because the pancreas does not respond appropriately. As a consequence of the sudden glucose drop (hypoglycemia), there is also a sudden feeling of hunger, and an absolute physical need to eat to provide some glucose to your brain. This bad cycle of inadequate eating habits starts again, exacerbated now by the insulin resistance of a pre-diabetic person.

The pre-diabetic situation can still be turned around by a diet and a change of lifestyle and habits. You *can* stop hurting your metabolism with constant glucose peaks. The 32 Mondays Weight Management Program and the associated lifestyle changes will lead to weight loss and, more specifically, to loss of belly fat. Remember that belly fat is your main enemy. You will learn in later chapters how belly fat also favors the production of the hormones that help you gain weight and are also directly related to prediabetes. If you don't turn the pre-diabetic situation around, over time your pancreas will tire from overproducing insulin, blood sugar will remain high for several hours after a meal, and type II diabetes will be diagnosed.[5]

KEY POINTS

›   Insulin is responsible for removing glucose from the bloodstream.

›   More glucose (high-glycemic carbohydrates) translates into more fat accumulation.

›   Fiber, fat, and proteins slow down the absorption of glucose. Always include them in each meal. Never eat high-glycemic foods alone.

›   Constantly eating high-glucose foods burns the pancreas.

›   Learn about GI and GL.

›   Be your pancreas's friend and maintain low and constant sugar levels in your bloodstream.

›   After a meal, wait three to four hours before eating again.

›   Exercise before meals if possible.

PRINCIPLE 9
LEARNING ABOUT OTHER HORMONES

Directly or indirectly, hormones are responsible partially or in total for many of your body's actions and reactions, such as mood changes, feelings, sexual attraction, metabolism, and growth. More relevant to our discussion, they are directly and highly related to weight gain and weight loss. Some people, even doctors, tend to blame hormones for all the negative situations happening in our bodies, including weight gain. Hormones per se don't cause the situation. Something else is behind the changes: the natural equilibrium of the hormones, which biologically have the ability to be in perfect equilibrium, is imbalanced.

There is always a reason for hormone imbalance. Sometimes, there is a sickness directly involved, or maybe a medication to treat another condition that could affect hormone balance. But most of the time, you create such an imbalance with simple yet poor life habits that interfere with your normal hormonal equilibrium.

Your body is an amazing machine where thousands of actions occur one after the other in perfect balance. It is incredible to observe how the body can still work even when it is submitted to external stress factors such as pollution, sun radiation, sleep deprivation, stress, pesticides, colorants, and many more. There are certain things you can't avoid in your daily life, like radiation caused by depletion of the ozone layer or pollution (although you could try to live in a cleaner environment). There are, however, other things you can avoid or at least minimize. **You can fully control all the products you ingest and use.**

Hormone activity depends on the molecular structure—the physical appearance—of the hormone. In some way or another, that structure interacts with other parts involved in a metabolic process, activating a response. Some of the pesticides, colorants, preservatives, and even prescription drugs interact directly or indirectly with the normal functioning of some hormones. They could change the shape of the hormone or occupy the space where the hormone has to act, or they can simply "distract" the normal functioning. The effects can be short-term or long-term, and the negative activity can accumulate over time. Any hormonal change can have a negative impact on your body. The more natural and more artificial-ingredient-free your nutrition is, the lower the chances of a negative interaction between the normal functioning of your hormones and those other substances.

> *Artificially sweetened, zero-calorie drinks also interact with the sugar-insulin equilibrium. The sweetener makes your body think you are ingesting sugar, so your pancreas releases insulin and activates the same mechanisms as if it was. In the end, a hunger response will be activated once the body realizes that after activating the metabolic mechanisms, there is nothing real to use as energy, so it claims the "real thing." In the short term, you are not ingesting calories directly, but in the long term, artificial sweeteners will disturb the sugar metabolism the same way as simple sugars, maybe even worse. Trying to curtail hunger by drinking those beverages will result in weight gain, either because of extra hunger, excessive storage caused by the inability to regulate our body fat mass, or lowered basic metabolism—the consumption of fewer calories by our bodies.*

When you switch to a natural diet and healthy lifestyle by eating and using toxin-free products instead of processed products full of preservatives, pesticides, and colorants that interact with your hormones, you will see an improvement in your overall health. You'll learn more in Step 14, but for now, just know that by doing so, you will achieve lower "bad" cholesterol levels and decreased blood pressure, lose weight, and enjoy healthier skin. This doesn't mean you can never eat prepackaged or even precooked meals, or have a conventional shampoo or skin-care product, but read the ingredients list to make sure there are not too many unnecessary and artificial ingredients, and try to use them as little as possible.

By now you have a good understanding of how complex the hormonal world is and therefore how important it is to balance its equilibrium. You also need to understand that all body mechanisms are interrelated; therefore, when managing hormonal aspects related to your weight management, remember that other factors like stress, happiness, sleep, and sex could also be involved. I would like to give you a general idea of the hormones that can be involved in your weight management so you are aware of them and pay special attention to them. We already considered insulin at length, so let's talk about the rest.

Human Growth Hormone

Human growth hormone (HGH) stimulates fat burning and helps muscle development, plus it strengthens your bones and reduces blood pressure. It also helps in the repair of cells and organs.

Its activity takes place at night when HGH "heals" your body. So, it is imperative that you get enough uninterrupted sleep. Also, to get all the energy the hormone requires for its activity, HGH (also known as growth hormone or GH) burns fat accumulated in your fat storage when there is no other energy available. That means if you are interested in burning fat, no free energy should be available for the hormone by the time you go to sleep. More about this in Step 13.

Practically speaking, you need to sleep at least seven hours for HGH to work. When and what you eat before going to sleep is also important. A dinner low in carbohydrates and rich in proteins activates HGH, so that's the ideal combination to eat a few hours before going to bed so all direct energy is already used up when you fall asleep. That way, HGH will reach out for the stored fat to use as an energy source.

On the other hand, when you have a dinner rich in carbohydrates just before bed and you don't sleep enough hours, you are inhibiting the action of your great ally, the growth hormone, and you're missing the fat burning associated with it.

Intense exercise (any exercise other than just walking, like strength training, running, biking, and swimming) stimulates HGH; therefore, exercising anytime in the evening is a smart option to get an additional help losing weight.

Adrenaline and Noradrenaline

Two other hormones, adrenaline and noradrenaline, help burn fat tissue. They are secreted when exercising and help provide the muscle with energy by burning stored fat. If you were looking for another reason to exercise, here you have it.

Leptin

Leptin is secreted by fat cells after a meal. This hormone sends a message to your brain indicating you are full. The leptin brain receptors suppress appetite signals so the body stops being hungry and starts burning calories. Therefore, when leptin works properly, it helps to reduce fat storage, but when it doesn't, your brain keeps asking for food because the hunger signals are on all the time.

When glucose levels are too low (from too many hours between meals or from skipping a meal) or after following restrictive diets, leptin is not secreted. Without leptin, you feel **an intense hunger and an unstoppable desire to eat**, especially carbohydrates, which is the brain's way of signaling a need for glucose.

The more fat cells you have, the more leptin you produce, but contrary to what you might think, leptin doesn't help you in your weight management mission. When you are overweight, it is for a reason, perhaps because you haven't paid too much attention to all the mechanisms and hormones that are telling you to stop eating. Well, leptin reacts in a manner similar to insulin. If you stimulate leptin production over the years by eating constantly, you can become leptin-resistant. Although levels of leptin are still high after a meal, its receptors no longer recognize it, so neuropeptide Y is never shut off and your sense of hunger is still "on." The fat-burning result never takes place.

When you lose some weight, your body recovers its sensitivity to leptin and its ability to control your hunger. Your body can then activate your fat-burning machine much easier.

Under restrictive dieting, your body thinks you are starving. It stops leptin production so you will feel hungry and *eat*. Poor sleep also decreases leptin levels.

Ghrelin

Your stomach secrets ghrelin to tell your brain you are hungry. When your body requires more nutrients, it secretes this hormone to make you aware of its needs and stays there until the needs are fulfilled. Once you have eaten, it takes a while until the mechanisms to stop ghrelin release come into action. That is the reason you always hear the recommendation to eat slowly. Slowing down your eating not only gives your digestive enzymes time to break down the food, but also to stop the feeling of hunger caused by ghrelin.

Ghrelin works to protect your body from famine. It is, therefore, very insistent and persuasive. Ghrelin is the one making you feel hungry, like sickly hungry, when your stomach is empty. Not that feeling of, umm, I would like to eat, but, *hey*, I am *starving*. Too much ghrelin is the reason I recommend you never skip a meal. Eat breakfast after the whole night of fasting, and eat a snack three to four hours after your proper meal.

A recent discovery[6] suggests ghrelin might also activate regions in your brain that make you desire food, like an obsession. Those regions look similar to the ones linked to drug addiction. So it is being suggested that food can also work as a sort of addiction.

If you maintain a diet low in calories, ghrelin levels are always high, and sooner or later this hormone will persuade you to eat wildly to cover your needs. You need to maintain ghrelin at low levels by eating enough at each meal and by snacking on healthy foods every three to four hours.

The only exception is at night, when HGH is released because its activity is favored by high ghrelin levels. By eating two to three hours before going to sleep, your stomach will be almost empty and HGH can rise and do its beneficial duty.

Cortisol

Cortisol is a stress hormone. Thinking you will never find a solution or that a particular situation will never end has negative repercussions in your body, and the cortisol released in those situations has something to do with it. Cortisol not only increases the cravings for high-carbohydrate and high-fat food, but it also lowers leptin—the hormone that tells you that you are not hungry anymore—and increases neuropeptide Y—the hormone that makes you rabidly hungry—thereby increasing your appetite.

Cortisol also favors the accumulation of fat in the abdominal area. And guess what: the more abdominal fat, the more cortisol released.

A positive outlook, a balanced diet high in protein, and plenty of quality sleep all help to keep cortisol levels under control.

Hormonal Changes When Aging

Estrogen levels in women change as we age (and more specifically, when we enter menopause) and these changes make it easier to gain weight. A woman's estrogen changes from one type to another: from the youth-type estradiol, which keeps your burning metabolism high and your fat storages under control, to the estrone form, which not only does exactly the opposite, but also moves your fat to your belly, which is the worst type of fat. Studies have shown that during menopause, the impaired estrogen signals may be the cause of the menopause weight gain.[7] Progesterone also drops, which causes a drop in its metabolic burning help.

Testosterone—a hormone essential for both men and women—is also a youth hormone, and we have less and less available while aging. Testosterone helps build muscle and burn fat, so as we add years, we not only add fat—especially abdominal fat—but we also lose muscle mass. And to make things worse, not only do our libidos slip as a consequence of less testosterone, but our motivation to exercise does, too. As we gain more weight, testosterone is converted to estrogen, the fattening one, which leads to more fat, which leads to more estrogen… see the pattern? Exercise stimulates testosterone production, so exercising more to compensate for the decrease in hormonal activity is a necessity as you age.

Aging doesn't work in your favor when it comes to hormones and weight management, but on the plus side, you have more experience: you know your body and your reactions to food, and how you react under stressful situations. By making all factors related to weight management work in your favor, you are better able to keep your weight under control. That's much easier if you continue exercising—even though it might require more persistence than when you were younger.

KEY POINTS

Hormones are responsible for regulating many functions in the human body. To be hormone friendly:

›   Eat a diet filled with whole, organic food, and avoid heavily processed food.

›   Several hormones are affected by sleep deprivation, so ensure you have a good night's sleep.

›   Eat a low-carbohydrate, high-protein dinner so your glucose levels are low and you secrete more ghrelin, which helps HGH do a proper job and help with your weight management tasks.

›   Don't go to bed with a full stomach because your HGH levels will be suppressed.

›   Exercise, especially at night, because you will activate HGH work.

›   Keep leptin and ghrelin levels balanced by eating every three to four hours.

›   Maintain a positive outlook and keep your generic stress levels under control to reduce cortisol production.

›   Keep exercising, especially as you age.

PRINCIPLE 10
UNDERSTANDING METABOLIC SYNDROME

Metabolic syndrome (MS) is *scary*. I left this discussion for you to read right before you start your 32 Mondays Weight Management Program so you don't forget about it. You might think you are far away from suffering from MS, but you could already have a few symptoms.

The IDF defines metabolic syndrome as a cluster of the most dangerous heart attack risk factors:

› diabetes and raised fasting plasma glucose

› abdominal obesity

› high "bad" cholesterol (LDL)

› high blood pressure

Two other conditions are also related to a diagnosis of metabolic syndrome:

› elevated triglycerides

› low "good" cholesterol (HDL)

People with metabolic syndrome are twice as likely to die and three times as likely to have a heart attack or stroke as the rest of the population.[8]

Experts are still investigating all the factors that play a role in developing metabolic syndrome, but the IDF has already determined the most important two causes for MS are insulin resistance and central obesity, which we've already looked at.

If you think you might already suffer from metabolic syndrome, or you'd like more information, you will find it at https://www.idf.org Assess all the symptoms, and determine if a visit to your doctor is mandatory to help address it.

KEY POINTS

› If you have three of the factors outlined, you could be diagnosed with metabolic syndrome, with its associated risks of heart attack and death.

› Losing weight, improving your diet, and increasing your exercise will help you manage metabolic syndrome.

You now have an understanding of the main principles behind many of the suggestions and recommendations I will give you in each of the 15 Steps of the 32 Mondays Weight Management Program. Keep the principles in mind, and come back to review them whenever I suggest you do so or when you think you have forgotten something.

Armed with your 10 Principles, you are now ready to rock the 15 Steps of the 32 Mondays Weight Management Program and change the way you manage your weight forever.

BEFORE YOU START: TREATS, DEVIATIONS, AND THE ART OF BALANCE

The most restrictive diets work against your weight management objective, which is to learn how to be in control of your physical, psychological, and emotional balance. As I said before, you can't follow a perpetual diet, program, or strict rule. That is the perfect recipe for failure. The time will come when you are tired, having a bad day and need a break, or just need to relax. Sometimes you are simply in a situation where you can't choose what to eat.

That is why it is not my intention for this program to be your jail guard, keeping the gates closed while you push to open them. You can't live against your interest and nature. The objective is to re-educate your way of eating, your habits, and your tastes slowly, step-by-step, to give you time to assimilate every change and enjoy your new way of eating until it feels just… right. That doesn't mean you always have to be so strict. You can't always live under rules.

We all need some freedom in our lives. Your body will undergo such a dramatic change after you follow this program that it will be able to compensate naturally for those small deviations. You will learn how to deal with parties and special occasions. I don't mean that after you finish this program you'll be able to cheat as much as you want without consequences… what I mean is that after this program, your body won't be craving and asking you to cheat that often because you won't be in a restrictive mode all the time, but will instead be in harmony and balance. When you come to those risky situations (let's say parties), you won't feel the need to jump into carbs because you won't be missing and craving them that much. So you'll be able to evaluate the situation, decide what you really want to eat, and reorganize the rest of the meal.

Once your body is in balance, it knows that it will always have enough food coming. If one day you eat too much, it will activate a burning mode to compensate. As I said before, that doesn't mean that you don't have to be careful in those special situations, but you don't need to be obsessed, which by the way does not help with weight management.

It is also okay to have one treat every day if you've eaten well that day.

Knowing that you can have a treat will allow you to relieve some pressure during the process of changing and maintaining your new habits. You just need to decide what your treat will be: a piece of chocolate, a candy, a cookie, a small ice-cream cone or waffle, some bacon, or a few chips perhaps? Then you need to be aware of its impact on your body, recognize it as a treat, and enjoy it!

Be aware of the effect on your body: For example, candy is direct sugar into your bloodstream, which means an insulin peak ahead. On the other hand, ice cream is mixed with some fat and therefore it is more fulfilling and produces a lower insulin reaction, but it is higher in calories than just sugar. Let's say you had a nice meal and you feel full, then avoid dessert! On the contrary, if you really behaved during dinner and had a light meal that was low in carbs, and maybe you are even hungry… go for the ice cream. The fat and protein from the milk will help you feel satisfied, which will get you through to the next meal (in three to four hours) and avoid snacking earlier.

Determine how often you are having those treats. Maybe you can have a small piece of chocolate every day, but ice cream or bacon only from time to time.

Sugary products should always come after a complete meal so they will mix with fats and proteins and have reduced absorption. Treats should always come **at the end of the day**. Knowing you have your small reward waiting will help you stay on track during the day. Never have your treat in the morning; after your good night's sleep and a healthy breakfast, your willpower is in full supply, so you are ready to make good decisions, and you won't need to use your small treat to keep you on the right path. The exception here would be something that isn't sweet, like bacon, which you could have over the weekend if you had a good week following the Steps. Weekends should give you a little bit of room for freedom to allow for some of the not-so-healthy choices.

Remember that by the end of the day, your ability to make the right decisions is diminished, so plan your treat ahead of time and stay with it. Do not leave the decision until the last minute.

If at some point you feel that you are getting off track more than you should, you need to come back to the 32 Mondays Weight Management

Program as soon as possible. Losing your focus is different from having a treat once in a while, and it will be more and more difficult to return to the right way the longer you wait to do it. It is never too late. Just start reviewing your food and exercise journals and each step again to see where you are slipping, and then get back on the right path.

We deserve the right to make mistakes while we work, study, raise our kids, take care of our elders, and feed ourselves. Overcoming your mistakes is essential to continuing on the right pathway with your life. If you fall deep into your guilt, determination to return to the right way takes longer. The same thing applies to a deviation on the pathway to healthy eating.

KEY POINTS

› Some treats are okay from time to time. There is no need to feel guilty if treating yourself is under control.

› Let the idea of a treat at night help get you through the day.

› Have your daily treat at night after your meal when you are sure you have behaved during the day.

› Come back to the right path as soon as possible if you are deviating too much.

PART II

32 MONDAYS WEIGHT MANAGEMENT PROGRAM'S 15 STEPS

Now that you understand the basics of the 32 Mondays Weight Management Program, you're ready to master its 15 Steps. Because the steps are interrelated, it is important that you read all of them once before starting the program so you understand them.

Suggested Time Frame

Each step can be an important change for you as you make the transition to your new, healthier lifestyle. I have established a specific amount of time for each step based on the difficulty of changing or adopting a new behavior and the associated challenges. There are two reasons you should respect the allocated time: first, because you need the time to understand and then learn and apply each step. Second, because the chance for success when changing two habits or behaviors at the same time is much lower than when you approach them one at a time. If a specific step is easier or more difficult for you, you might need less or more time than what I suggest, and that's okay. If you are positive that you have already mastered that step, go ahead and move on to the next one. If you think you need more time, go ahead and take it. Just make sure that you are not procrastinating about adopting the changes you need to make.

STEP	NAME	TIMING (Weeks)
1	Eat Less Every Meal	2
2	Start Moderate Exercise	1
3	Drinks	2
4	Composition and Organization of Meals	2
5	Snacking	2
6	Fats	4
7	Sugars	4
8	Carbohydrates	4
9	Salt	1
10	Alcohol	1
11	Vigorous Exercise	4
12	Fruits and Vegetables	2
13	Sleep	1
14	Go Organic	1
15	Be Happy for the Rest of Your Life	1

STEP 1
EAT LESS EVERY MEAL

SUGGESTED TIME FRAME: 2 WEEKS

In this first step, you'll begin eating less. You will not lose an enormous amount of weight, but you are setting the basis for steady weight loss, a bit every week. When added to the rest of the steps, this will help you lose weight in the long run and, most important, forever.

You probably are accustomed to eating more than your body needs. As usual, there is not only one explanation for that.

You don't eat just to satisfy hunger: you also eat because food tastes good. Food has become more refined, more palatable, more appealing, and that's made it difficult to learn to stop eating when your stomach is full. If you had just a few simple things to eat, but you could eat as much as possible, you would eat much less. That's part of the reason for the success of the diets that let you eat as much as you want but restrict the variety of foods. You get bored, you eat less, and you end up losing weight. That is, until you have all the food available again. Then you start to eat too much of the food you like, and you regain the weight you lost.

Begin today to reprogram your mind to understand that all food is always available, and you need to take only what you really need. You don't need to be hungry when you leave the table. You need to feel as if maybe you would eat more, but you can manage without it. To be able to do that, you need to start with small portions to calculate how much you need. If you start with a huge plate of food, you'll find it is difficult to throw away what should be left. It is much easier to start with a small serving and add little portions if necessary.

Always think in advance what you are planning to include in a meal. If you plan to eat a piece of fruit and a small piece of chocolate or a cookie at the end of the meal, you need room for that. That means your portions of chicken, pasta, and other parts of your meal need to be small enough to have room left for your treat without overeating. You need the vitamins from the fruit, and it is really difficult to say no when you planned for that cookie, so leave room for it!

Now, the reality is that for one reason or another, you eat too much and exercise too little. This is a *big truth*: **You always underestimate how much you eat and overestimate how much you exercise.** An important reason for this is a lack of understanding about average serving sizes.

This is what an *average serving size* looks like:

›   **Salad**: two hands together = 1 cup

›   **Lean meat, poultry, and fish**: size and thickness of the center of your palm = 4 ounces (110 grams)

›   **Cheese, salad dressing, oil, seeds, hummus, guacamole**: two thumbs = 2 tablespoons of liquid or 1 ounce (30 grams)

›   **Nuts**: two thumbs or about 14 walnuts, 18 cashews, 20 hazelnuts or pistachios, 33 peanuts

›   **Vegetables, milk, fruit, yogurt, beans, legumes**: one fist-size portion = 1 cup or 7 ounces (200 grams)

›   **Carbohydrates (cereal, pasta, rice, couscous, quinoa)**: 1 cup or 7 ounces (200 grams), 1 medium slice of bread.

A special note about carbohydrates: limit your serving size to one cup or slice! We tend to serve and eat double this portion size!

If you are a larger person, your serving sizes might need to be increased.

If you exercise a lot, your serving sizes, especially protein, might need to be larger, too.

Menu Templates

For the next two weeks, reduce the amount of food according to the template below. Depending on your size and activity level, this is the amount of food you should be eating. I know you probably won't be there in two weeks, but that is your goal. The objective is to be there once you finish the 32 Mondays Weight Management Program. And remember, your best ally is your food diary. Keeping it will help you recognize what you have eaten during the day, and you can go back to check what you have been doing if you aren't obtaining your expected results.

> › Breakfast:
>> ○ 1 serving milk, yogurt, or cheese
>> ○ 1 serving whole grain bread, pasta, oats, or low-sugar cereal with high-fiber protein
>> ○ ½ serving of protein: meat or one egg
>> ○ Coffee or tea (see note)
>
> › Morning snack:
>> ○ 1 serving nuts, cheese, yogurt, or hummus
>> ○ ½ serving cereal, fruit, vegetables or ½ avocado
>
> › Lunch:
>> ○ 1 serving salad or vegetables
>> ○ 1 serving pasta, whole grain bread, or other carb
>> ○ 1 serving meat, fish, egg, tofu,* or other protein
>> ○ 1 serving fruit or yogurt

> › Afternoon snack:

> > ○ 1 serving nuts, cheese, yogurt, or hummus

> > ○ ½ serving cereal, fruit, vegetables, or whole grain bread or ½ avocado

> › Dinner:

> > ○ 1 serving salad or vegetables

> > ○ 1 serving meat, fish, egg, tofu,* or other protein

> > ○ 1 serving fruit or yogurt

> > ○ 1 treat

> > ○ ***No carbs at night!***

(*) Tofu or bean curd is a food derived from coagulated soy milk. It is a food rich in vegetarian protein.

Note: If you like coffee or tea with milk or cream, use the respective serving size. And if you use sugar, reduce the amount of carbs in your breakfast until you learn how to drink your coffee or tea unsweetened. If you use artificial sweeteners, reduce the amount until you are able to quit them.

The objective of this menu plan template is to help you eat the recommended serving sizes and not be hungry. It is specifically designed so your blood sugar levels are in equilibrium during the day; you won't have huge insulin peaks so you won't have cravings, especially for carbs, and you won't be hungry until it is time for your next meal.

If your dinner is really early, you should substitute the afternoon snack for the nighttime snack, or save part of the afternoon snack and part of dinner to eat as a nighttime snack. Organize your meals according to your personal and family schedules. You will learn more about this in Steps 4 and 5.

Practical Tips to Help You Eat Less

The reality is that you need fewer calories than you are eating right now; One reason is because you are eating without awareness; the other is the too-large portions you are used to. Accept these facts and be ready to change. ***Remember to control your serving sizes and list everything you eat in your food diary.***

To avoid mindless eating, you need to pay attention. Plan your meals knowing how many times you will eat that day, which meal you are about to have, and what is included in each meal. Eat seated and be mindful of what you are putting in your mouth. More about this in Step 4.

Remember, it takes about twenty minutes for your brain to receive the signal that makes you realize you are full. So, eat slowly and pay attention to how you feel, and stop as soon as you realize you are full. Remember the paradigm about the French—they are thin despite the amount of butter and cheese they eat. Something else is at work here: they eat calmly, sitting down and enjoying every bit of their food. The moment they changed this eating habit by eating a fast-food meal, they began to gain weight.

Have a snack three to four hours after each meal to avoid extreme hunger when you get to the table for your next meal. Eat calmly, slowly, and let your brain signal when you've had enough.

Choose satisfying foods that make you feel full, including fats and protein in each meal, to let you enjoy each and every meal, which will make these changes easier.

Here are some additional tips to help you:

> › Use smaller plates, bowls, and cutlery. Visual cues have an obvious impact on the amount our brain expects and therefore, on the amount you eat.

> › Never eat from the box. Prepare your portions in an appealing presentation before you feel hungry.

> › Start your meals with a light soup, a salad, or some vegetables. These

will fill you up without adding too many calories and will help you eat smaller portions of your main course.

› Drink a whole glass of water before each meal (8 oz. or approximately 250 ml.).

› Eat slowly. Studies[9,10] show that you will feel full and eat less food this way.

› Serve everyone's plate and then put the leftovers away.

› Always check serving sizes when checking food labels. You might find the serving size is very small so is the amount of calories you'll consume is too large to be worth it. You could choose another food option with a larger portion size so you feel more satiated.

Last Word

Counting calories is hard work and an unrewarding task, especially for the people who suffer from a lack of time—and that's most of us, right? I have no intention of asking you to count calories, but some idea of the numbers can help you a lot.

Did you know that even though a whole juicy apple has almost twice the calories of a rice cake, the glycemic index of the apple is 38 but the rice cake is 77?

Get into the habit of learning the calories, glycemic index, and glycemic load of foods you eat, and keep a list of those on hand for your favorites. This will help you organize your meals with those values in mind.

SUGGESTED TIME FRAME

Accomplishing this first step can be an important change for you. Constantly remind yourself about eating less at each meal to obtain maximum results. This is not difficult, but it does require attention all the time. This is why I allowed two weeks for this first step.

⤺

Congratulations! After two weeks, you probably have already lost some weight, and you are now in the routine of eating less in each meal. It's time to move forward to Step 2, which will help you lose weight even faster by starting moderate exercise.

TAKE 5

› **Learn**: Understand how to eat less.

› **Goal**: Eat only what is necessary to maintain your needs, following the recommended serving sizes and the suggested menu templates.

› **Plan**: Organize your meals according to serving sizes and personal menus.

› **Monitor**: Keep a food journal.

› **Reward**: Treat yourself to a book about calories, glycemic index, or of healthy recipes.

KEY POINTS

› You underestimate how much you eat and overestimate how much you exercise.

› Follow the template to eat less and control portion sizes.

› Pay special attention to the serving sizes, especially for carbohydrates.

› Keep a food diary to monitor your actual intake.

› Preplan your meals.

› Follow the menu templates to avoid feeling hungry.

STEP 2
START MODERATE EXERCISE

SUGGESTED TIME FRAME: 1 WEEK

Now that you are eating less at every meal, you also need to establish the habit of leading an active lifestyle. Exercise has plenty of benefits, and without any doubt the most important are feeling better, losing weight, balancing your hormones, and improving your mood. This is essential to be able to keep pursuing each of the 15 Steps.

There is no need yet to start intense exercise—that will come later, once you have mastered other basic principles and dropped some weight so you can move your body more freely.

After starting a moderate exercise routine, you won't see a huge weight drop, but as in the previous step, it will help you drop small amounts of weight daily and forever without even being aware that you're doing so. How are you ever going to incorporate changes into your life and eating habits if you feel negative and have a bad temper? On the contrary, when you feel positive and happy, you can see how easy it can be to change certain things. When you start to see yourself as an active person, you will feel motivated to adopt the other steps you have ahead.

From the physiological point of view, moderate exercise increases metabolism, improves circulation, and helps regulate your body processes.

Merriam-Webster defines metabolism as "the chemical changes in living cells by which energy is provided for the vital processes and activities and new material is assimilated to repair the waste."[11] This is what happens inside your body in terms of cell and organ activity that makes your body work properly. When you increase your metabolism by exercising, you increase the need for energy for that exercise. When you increase the energy requirements, your body either has to use the immediate energy you have just consumed—that apple you had for a snack—or if there is nothing directly available, the body burns fat and liberates its energy. Exercise also helps balance the human growth factor hormone that helps you with weight management, endorphins that help combat stress and anxiety and therefore reduce the production of excess cortisol, the stress hormone that makes us search for food; and finally, adrenaline and noradrenaline, which help burn fat to provide energy.

Moderate exercise is not going to make you slim. Not even strenuous exercise will do that. (We discuss muscle development, endorphins, and high metabolism in Step 11.) It takes about twenty minutes of light swimming or walking to burn a simple apple! But just thirty minutes of any type of exercise increases your metabolism. It might not burn that apple immediately, but it leaves the body in a state that continues burning calories for a while. When you move from a sedentary lifestyle into an active one, your body is in burning mode. It is always burning what it has available. If your metabolism is activated, it works twenty-four hours a day in your favor. That means the extra sugar you had this morning, which required additional insulin, won't be there. That sugar was used when choosing the stairs instead of the elevator, so the sugar won't be stored. Although you didn't burn that specific apple after just a walk, you helped your weight management in a much greater way. This is not just about how many calories you burn, but what is going on in your body.

Don't Overdo It at the Gym

You've already learned new eating habits that lead you, no doubt, to have more energy without increasing your caloric intake. When you follow the 32 Mondays Weight Management Program, you will have extra energy for an active lifestyle. When you exercise moderately you tone both large and small muscles. Muscles burn far more calories than simple fat (more about this in Step 11).

When I see overweight people at my gym working with a trainer who forces them into heavy weight lifting and strenuous running, it breaks my heart. They suffer so much and try so hard that I wish I had the courage to talk to them and convince them to follow this Program and only start vigorous exercise after they lose enough weight to feel lighter and more flexible. They appear so tired when they finish, and they probably realize that after so much effort, there isn't a big difference to see. Not only that, but they have probably no stamina left to pursue any other challenge, like eating less and better, organizing the right meals, or cooking a healthy meal after the gym visit.

Really, if you have a significant amount of weight to lose, go through this Program practicing moderate exercise until you lose some weight. Use the additional energy and motivation you've gained to visit the grocery store, choose the right products, and cook some healthy, light, and yummy meals for the rest of the week.

Ladies, you are most likely killing yourself in the gym trying to reduce your butt, thighs, or stomach. You should first focus on following this Program until you change the way you eat. I can assure you that you will see a change in your body. Please wait until you arrive at Step 11 for vigorous exercise; that's when you should start to focus directly on the body parts you specifically want to improve.

Practical Ways to Increase Moderate Exercise

Moderate exercise is easy, free, and inexpensive. You don't need to belong to an expensive gym or purchase a lot of equipment to enjoy the benefits of raising your metabolism. Some of the activities you can do include walking, light swimming, biking, or simply taking the stairs instead of the elevator. Let's focus on the two I find are easiest for most people: walking and moderate water exercise.

Walking

The first great, easy, fun (and free!) exercise anyone can ever do is walking. There are no limits for walking. You can go by yourself, with friends, or with your dog. You can walk in the woods, the city, the gym, or the mountains. You can listen to the news, music, your friend, or you can simply think and observe. You can be old or young. And if it is cold, you will burn extra calories by generating heat to protect yourself against the cold.

Although walking is relatively simple, it is important to practice good habits so you get the most benefit from your walking time. Always try to maintain a straight posture. Keep your abdominal muscles tight, so you not only work your abdominals, but also maintain a healthy back. Contract your legs and buttocks to develop the muscles in that area (we all want a nice, tight butt and legs). Every little bit you do makes a difference!

The beauty of walking is that it can be done virtually anywhere by almost anyone. If you use public transportation, leave some extra time and exit the bus one or two stops before your usual one. If you're driving, park a bit farther away from your destination than you usually do.

Miss your friend? You can ask him or her to join you for a walk every day. If you struggle to find time to get together, try early in the morning or late at night if you are busy during the day, or while the kids are at school if you are a homemaker.

Miss your partner? Try to have a nice walk with him or her every day to talk about your day instead of sitting in front of the TV while eating something inappropriate. Not only will your weight management improve, but so will your relationship.

By yourself? Take the opportunity to listen to the news or some music using any of the devices available today. Search a bit and you'll find there is something perfect for your needs and your budget. Or just think while you walk! That's something we never seem to have enough time to do.

Need to take care of the kids? Hire a neighbor babysitter for an hour. You'll find plenty of them willing to babysit for a short period of time, and it will be money well spent—not only for your weight, but also for your mind (time away from your kids for a while), your partner (if you decide to go with him or her), your friendship (if you go with a friend), your dog (who will be delighted with that extra walk), and your kids: they will learn the importance of a healthy lifestyle and will learn to respect your need for some free time to exercise.

How Much Should You Walk?

You can invest a few dollars in a pedometer, a small device you wear that measures how many steps you are taking per day. The pedometer senses your body motion and counts your footsteps. The count is converted into distance by knowing the length of your usual stride. You can always get one of the fancy watches or applications if they are useful to you. But remember, no matter how good your equipment or app is, it won't exercise for you! You are the one who has to do the work.

A pedometer can help you determine how sedentary or active you are. From this starting point, you can determine how much you should increase your daily low-impact activity. You can wear the pedometer all day and record total steps. As a reference, Dr. Catrine[12] Tudor-Locke recommends the following, which is based on research:

Classification of Pedometer-Determined Physical Activity in Healthy Adults

- *Less than 5,000 steps/day may be considered a "sedentary lifestyle index."*

- *5,000–7,499 steps/day is typical of daily activity, excluding sports/exercise, and might be considered "low active."*

- *7,500–9,999 steps/day likely includes some exercise or walking (and/or a job that requires more walking) and might be considered "somewhat active."*

- *10,000 steps/day indicates the point that should be used to classify individuals as "active."*

- *Individuals who take more than 12,500 steps/day are likely to be classified as "highly active."*

I suggest you do at least thirty minutes of light exercise per day, which means approximately two thousand to three thousand *additional* steps per day if your exercise is walking. If you are sedentary right now, start with a slow pace, but set an objective of increasing it every week. You can wear your pedometer when you go out for a walk as a motivation tool to know how much you are doing in the same interval of time.

Once you are able to maintain a faster pace, try interval walking by increasing your pace to a maximum for a few seconds. You will increase your metabolism and fat-burning process, too.

By the way, buy a good pair of walking or even running shoes (looking to the future) to help your hips and joints.

Water Exercises

If you like the water and you have access to a pool, pool walking and exercising are also excellent mild to moderate exercises. Water cushions the exercise so it's easy on your joints and hips, but at the same time, it requires more effort than the same activity on land because you have to go against the force of the water. Have you ever tried a water aerobic group session or something similar? You'll need to join a gym for this, and you can ask there which moderate-intensity classes are available. They'll be able to help you find the class that's right for you. It is fun, less intense than swimming or water aerobics, and you'll be surprised to see how many people enroll in those sessions; you might even find a new exercise partner.

Incorporating Moderate Exercise into Daily Life

Every small increase of activity counts. One of the reasons you can't lose weight is because you don't have enough daily activity. Don't gain extra weight by doing less and less on a daily basis—try these ideas instead:

> › Found your old bicycle? Try some light cycling around the block and run some errands.

> › Have stairs at home, at work, anywhere? Use them as much as possible. You are not only increasing your exercise but also rounding your buttocks!

> › Have kids or dogs or both? They'll love running and playing with you. Instead of merely watching them play, get involved in the game.

> › Love gardening? Plan on planting and trimming as much as possible to have a wonderful garden.

> › Have a lawn? Get rid of the mowing company and do it yourself. It is not only good exercise, but it will save you some cash to invest in organic food.

> › Go shopping with your friend or do any other activity that makes you move off your cozy sofa.

> › Contract your buttocks and abdominal muscles while sitting at the computer, driving, waiting for an appointment, or standing in line at school, the store, or anywhere you're normally sedentary.

Take a "Time Out"

No matter what your beliefs or your credo, you are probably familiar with the concept of stress and how bad it is for your body. Maybe your doctor already talked to you about this, or you know somebody whose health is taking a toll from too much stress. You can approach stress in various ways, but the moment you start moderate exercise, you'll be in the right path, as exercise is an excellent tool to reduce stress.

But apart from exercise, you also need some time every day to connect with yourself. I am not only talking about free time to do what you love to do, like hobbies, reading, or listening to music. I am talking about five minutes a day just for you, with nothing else taking place, to connect with yourself. Some time where you look inside yourself, see where you are, and let things inside you just flow. Your inner energy has an enormous power over what happens to you. It is also very wise. If you let it go, not interfering too much, it will lead you in the right direction. If you block it, it will push some way or another to get out, creating a negative effect somewhere in your body. You need a few minutes every day to stop your life and to listen to what is going inside, to make sure you are not stopping the natural energy flowing in your body. You stop, listen, and reconnect. With this tiny step, you can make sure you are heading in the right direction toward feeding your body the appropriate way, exercising, and having a healthy lifestyle. It helps you clear your mind, understand the messages for the right directions better, assimilate them, and act with a clear purpose.

Is this all new for you? You might find some inspiration at *http://meditationsociety.com/*.

Finding Time to Take a "Time Out"

Some excellent moments to reconnect with yourself are in bed right after waking up or before going to sleep. Take advantage of the bus or train ride. Maybe you have a few minutes while waiting somewhere, like a doctor's appointment, your daughter's ballet lesson, a conference call, or a business appointment. After exercising, when you are already relaxed, is one of the best moments of the day. Try the steam room or hot tub in your gym if you have one.

Just sit, close your eyes, let go of the overcharged energy in your body. Listen and feel what is running through your body; be thankful for what you have and for getting the vision and light to find the right way, and let go! If that sounds too basic to you, get a deeper understanding. I like the tips and explanations given at the New York Insight Meditation Center's website at https://www.nyimc.org/how-to-meditate/.

SUGGESTED TIME FRAME

You should be done with this step in one week. You don't need to understand complex information; you just need to do it. You might want to buy a pair of running shoes over the weekend or call a friend or a babysitter. You have one week to make the arrangements and start including moderate exercise in your life!

TAKE 5

› **Learn**: Understand how and why it is important to exercise and how you can increase your activity level.

› **Goal**: Practice moderate exercise daily for at least thirty minutes per day.

› **Plan**: Decide what your daily moderate exercise routines will be and when you will exercise.

› **Monitor**: Maintain an exercise journal.

› **Rewards**: Buy yourself a pedometer.

KEY POINTS

› Moderate activity increases your metabolism and well-being.

› Begin today!

› Determine which type of exercise is the best option for you.

› Go alone, with a friend, your dog, your kids, your partner, or find a group.

› Get a pedometer as a reward and monitor your daily steps.

› Practice "time out" to reconnect your mind and body and let your inner energy flow.

STEP 3
DRINKS

SUGGESTED TIME FRAME: 2 WEEKS

You have been eating less at each meal for two weeks and have been exercising moderately for one week. Feeling great? Let's have a look now at what you drink.

Drinks to Avoid

Unfortunately, if you are used to drinking sodas and/or other drinks all day long, it is going to be difficult not only to change your habits, but also to break the addiction that sugar and artificial sweeteners create in your body. The more you are used to drinking, the more difficult it will be to stop.

Not only are sugar and sweeteners addictive, but also the constant ingestion of them creates a peak in insulin that demands more and more sugar. This is exactly the same mechanism as nicotine, which is believed to be one of the most addictive substances. Sugar hasn't been declared an addictive drug yet, but it should be—it is addictive both physically and mentally. The good thing is that sugar and sweeteners are far less addictive and therefore much easier to overcome. Once you can control the physical addiction by not consuming the sugary or artificially sweetened drink, you are only left with the habit or psychological addiction.

Therefore, I suggest you cut the consumption of those drinks completely to stop the sugar/sweetener addiction right away. (If you are familiar with smoking-cessation programs, you will find the most effective ones are those that have you stop smoking completely and immediately to stop the nicotine addiction.)

Start drinking plain water and add some lemon or orange peels if desired. This way, you will be able to control the psychological need and habit of having something in your hand and drinking all the time. Invest in a fancy water bottle and always carry it with you.

Sugary Drinks

Are you are used to constantly drinking sodas or similar sugary drinks?

The bad news is that you *really* need to stop drinking them. The sugar contained in a can of soda is almost the daily total amount of sugar recommended by the World Health Organization (WHO) and has more calories than two apples or two slices of bread. Not only are you consuming empty calories compared to any healthy food you could be eating, but sugary drinks also feed pure sugar to your body. Do you remember how bad sugar is when trying to manage insulin and other related hormones? Sugary drinks punch your pancreas to overproduce insulin. In addition, if you usually drink sodas alone or between meals, you double the negative effects.

The good news is that as soon as you stop consuming sugary drinks, you will enjoy weight loss, an increase in your energy levels, a better mood, and an improvement in your general well-being.

If you are a moderate consumer of sugary drinks, you still need to consider how bad they are for you and how little they help you in your weight management and health improvement. Those drinks don't give you anything except pure sugar right into your bloodstream. You'll do yourself a big favor by not drinking sugary drinks and instead having real food packed with minerals, vitamins, and fiber. Any fresh fruit is an excellent substitute for a sugary drink.

Consider this: one can of soda contains 40 grams of sugar, or about ten sugar cubes. That is the equivalent of:

› 65 medium strawberries,

› 2 medium apples,

› ½ pineapple,

› 13 carrots,

› 7 plain Greek yogurts,

› 1 large bar of dark chocolate, or

› 3 servings of ice cream.

And if you're thinking about moving to low-calorie sodas… *don't do it.*

Low or Zero-Calorie Drinks

As you already know, the food and beverage industry is smart. It creates new and artificial needs that you end up believing are true needs.

When sugary drinks were getting bad press and people started avoiding them, the beverage industry invented zero-calorie drinks. This sounded perfect: you could maintain the addiction without adding calories to your diet. During the last two decades, the taste of zero- and low-calorie drinks have improved, and more and more flavors have been invented to cover all types of tastes.

Here is the bad news: although you thought they were harmless, they are far from that—not just for you but also for your children. Not only have some artificial sweeteners been demonstrated to be harmful to our health (causing arthritis, gastrointestinal problems, even cancer, among others), but they also interfere with sugar metabolism and increase your sugar cravings.[13]

When the artificial sweetener reaches your body, a signal is sent to the brain, which expects "sweet calories" to enter your body. When no calories are detected, the brain sends the hormonal message to ask for more calories since there were none. Not only that, but if you ingest too much sweetener (sweet without calories), your body forgets that sweets usually have lots of calories. Therefore, when you have a real sweet, your metabolism does not take any extra measures to burn those extra calories. You also desensitize your taste, and therefore you end up needing really sweet stuff to feel sweetly satisfied. That's a lot, right? Well, there is still more.

Sweeteners may also stimulate your appetite directly by making you secrete insulin when detecting unreal but "sweet" molecules. Insulin removes the real glucose you have in your bloodstream, and when you have low glucose levels, you feel hunger cravings that stimulate your appetite and make you look for food.

Recent research shows the consumption of low- or zero-calorie drinks increases the waistline in people, especially in women, even when not increasing their total weight.[14]

This doesn't mean you can never drink a soda or a low-calorie drink again, but just be aware of what you are giving your body and the insulin effect on it every time you drink one. By the way, stevia is a very concentrated natural sweetener. Since it is natural, it does not appear to have the potential harm of artificial sweeteners, although it is still too early to know since there is not enough conclusive research yet. But it is still a sweetener, so it does have the same impact on your metabolism as artificial sweeteners so try to avoid it as much as possible.

Drinks to Have in Moderation

I often hear people complain that drinking just water is boring. While it doesn't have to be (more about water in a moment), other beverage choices are available for occasional consumption.

Juices

Some people don't drink sugary or sweetened drinks, but they do drink fruit juices, with no added sugar, of course. Although fruit juices are packed with plenty of vitamins and even minerals, you also need to be careful with juices.

They still have all the sugar from the fruit —which can be a lot of sugar—but without the fiber of the whole piece of fruit. Fiber helps to retain the amount of free sugar in the bloodstream and thus lower the alarm for the pancreas to secrete insulin. So when drinking juices without that fiber, you generate an insulin response almost as strong as with any other sugary drink, and the response is even stronger when you drink the juice alone with no other food.

Also, because juices are tasty and easy to drink (compared to a whole piece of fruit), they are easy to drink in excess.

Note that packaged fruit juices also contain preservatives, which break the liquid homeostasis (equilibrium) in your intestine, sometimes causing diarrhea when you have them in excess. Be careful, especially with kids.

Kids are usually the family members who ingest insane volumes of fruit juices. Once they are used to them, it is difficult for kids to stop drinking juices. You need to explain why they are not that healthy. Kids can still have them, just not all the time. You can also switch to small juice boxes, especially for school lunches and away-from-home snacking, which still offer some satisfaction but have much less volume.

So please, limit the amount juice you drink, and always drink home-made juices or at least those with no added sugar (fruit already has enough sugar). If possible, add the pulp of the fruit to the juice. A serving of commercial orange juice with no sugar added contains 24 grams of sugar. Although it is healthier than a soda, it is still a lot of sugar without the fiber to slow down the absorption. Tomato juice is a great option since it contains a low amount of sugar (9 grams).

Sport Beverages and Energy Drinks

Another great invention by the food and beverage industry to boost sales was sports drinks. A few decades ago our grandparents gave us water with lemon and sugar after a great physical effort, but we now have a selection of sport beverages to choose from—drinks to consume before exercising, immediately after, after a few hours, to recover sugar, to develop muscles, with sugar and without it, with protein, and all the exotic flavors and colors of the world!

How many of us exercise enough to need any of those beverages?

Typically, only professional athletes and people exercising for a long period of time, especially in the heat (like my husband does), need them. In those situations, a specific drink full of minerals and electrolytes to help retain water and avoid dehydration is not only recommended but necessary. Other than some specific situation, all those drinks have the same effects as any soda or juice. Instead of a drink packed with corn starch, egg, corn syrup, caffeine, and other crazy ingredients, wouldn't it better to plan ahead and have a nice breakfast including an egg, some bread, and coffee or a lunch or snack that includes some protein, fats, and carbohydrates?

If we do use sports drinks to supplement workouts, we usually have them during or after exercise, thereby providing sugar to our bodies instead of letting them first burn the available sugar and then the glycogen and stored fat.

Energy drinks are popular today not only among people who exercise. I see average people at the grocery store buying cases of energy drinks and giving them to their children. And you know what? Something must be wrong because the only time I gave my daughter a blue energy drink, the color of her stools was *blue*! And I know that my kids are not the only ones. I don't think this is a specific problem with blue colors or with my daughter. Those drinks contain so many artificial colors and flavors that they can't do any good. Our metabolisms are not designed to deal with so many artificial products, so the less anyone has them—especially kids who are still developing—the better.

Having said that, if you need drinks to help you complete your exercise routines, or electrolytes for when is too hot or because you tend to be low in potassium and magnesium (like I am), make sure your drinks are sugar-, artificial sweetener-, color- and preservative-free.

Milk

As long as you aren't lactose intolerant, go for it! But remember that milk is not calorie-free or sugar-free, so count it and add it to your food journal. The benefit of drinking milk is that you'll be getting calcium. Some doctors and researchers opine that a high daily consumption of dairy products helps you lose weight, although it is not clear why; it could help release fat-burning hormones and enzymes, but that effect has not been studied deeply yet. Milk can also be a great substitute for your old drinks, but it should be reduced fat or fat free, and plain milk please, no chocolate or vanilla-sweetened milk, and no added sugar. You don't need the extra calories from the fat or the extra sugar. And for school or work lunches and snacks, individual milk packages are as convenient as juice boxes.

Coffee

If you drink coffee, make it plain and unsweetened if possible. The difference between a plain coffee and a Frappuccino is 250 calories. If you add whipped cream, you are ingesting as many calories and as much saturated fat as you would in a cheeseburger. Avoid nondairy creamers filled with chemicals. Have fat-free milk or nothing in your coffee. Getting used to unsweetened coffee is just a matter of practice. Stevia does not contain calories, and although it is natural, it is still a sweetener, and therefore it triggers your brain to react the same way artificial sweeteners do.

The hypothesis that caffeine is an ally for weight loss is being studied, but nothing conclusive has yet been decided, and caffeine abuse won't help you with your sleep, blood pressure, or other issues. So make it your choice, but don't abuse it if you choose caffeine.

Tea and Herbs

As with coffee, drink teas unsweetened. I assure you that you can do it! If you really can't avoid sugar, use as little as possible.

I consider all types of teas and herbs the same. Although there is some consideration that some types of teas and herbs help with weight loss, there is no scientific-based data that corroborates the statement, so I can't support it. On the other hand, people tend to think that because herbs are natural they are harm-free. Well, natural herbs can be as harmful as a medication, so make sure you learn what are you having before drinking it just in case it is not as safe as you think.

Water: The Healthiest Drink

Nothing is better for you than drinking water. It gives you a sense of fullness and therefore less of a sense of hunger, which is useful right before your meals. Water hydrates your body and returns the water to your skin for that beautiful, glowing aspect. Water helps eliminate toxins from your body and helps your body function properly. Sometimes you mistake hunger for thirst, so when you feel hungry, always have a glass of water first. This is applicable for everybody but especially for children. You'd be surprised at how many kids suffer health consequences from not drinking enough water. Sometimes, kids may even reach dehydration or suffer from low blood pressure and fainting spells when they don't consume a sufficient amount of water.[15]

One of the best things you can do to increase your weight loss and help your body function optimally is to replace any drink you were having with six to eight glasses of water (about 1.5 to 1.7 liters) per day.

Tips for Increasing Water Intake

- *Carry a water bottle with you always, no matter where you go. Drink every now and then until you finish it, even if you don't feel thirsty.*

- *Keep a small glass of water in the kitchen and drink it every time you see it.*

- *Keep a bottle of water by your bed and drink before you go to sleep and right after you wake up.*

- *Avoid waiting to drink until you are thirsty. Once you are thirsty, you are already suffering the initial effects of dehydration.*

- *Always drink a glass of water right before your meals to fill up your stomach a bit and make you feel fuller with less food.*

- *Try adding lemon, cucumber, and mint to a jar of water and refrigerate it for a few hours, and then enjoy it! You can fill up the jar four or five times until the mint gets old.*

SUGGESTED TIME FRAME

I have allowed two weeks for this step, not because it is difficult to understand and apply, but because of the addiction aspect of sugar and other drinks. If you are used to them, you will need the first week to break your sugar addiction (withdrawal from a physical addiction to nicotine also takes one week). More time will be required to break the psychological habit of drinking sodas and other sweetened drinks. It might take you more than two weeks to forget about drinking them and to feel comfortable with your new choices, but you need to set up a time line to advance and achieve your goal. Two weeks should be enough. Even if you don't drink sugary sweetened drinks, you might need these two weeks to remove sugar from your coffee or tea or to get used to drinking six to eight glasses of water per day.

TAKE 5

›   **Learn**: Understand how sugary and sweetened drinks interfere with your metabolism and make you fat.

›   **Goal**: Avoid sugary and sweetened drinks.

›   **Plan**: Know when you desire more sugary drinks and get ready with a glass of water or a non-sugary, unsweetened drink.

›   **Monitor**: Follow your improvements in the food journal.

›   **Reward**: Treat yourself with a super cool water bottle.

KEY POINTS

›   Sugary drinks are addictive.

›   Sugary drinks activate insulin peaks and reduce the glucose levels suddenly, causing subsequent food cravings.

› Zero-calorie or sugar-free drinks have a negative effect on your metabolism by:

  ○ activating insulin peaks,

  ○ activating cravings when no real sugar is present, making you feel hungry,

  ○ causing you to lose a sense of how sweet real sugar is, and

  ○ making your waistline larger.

› Juices have a lot of sugar with no fiber from the fruit to reduce sugar absorption.

› Sport beverages should only be consumed if you need to recover the electrolytes you have lost during a workout. That will be the case if you had an intense session (at least thirty minutes of intense exercise) or you sweat a lot. Again, be careful with your choices so you only add electrolytes and not sugar or artificial flavors and colors.

› Drink milk without added sugar and count it in the food diary.

› Drink coffee and tea with nonfat milk only—avoid nondairy creamers.

› Learn to drink coffee and tea without sugar or artificial or natural sweeteners.

› Drink six to eight glasses of water per day.

STEP 4
COMPOSITION AND ORGANIZATION OF MEALS

SUGGESTED TIME FRAME: 2 WEEKS

This is one of your most important steps, and, to me, it's one of the easier ones, as you don't need to make big changes—just apply a bit of reorganization and planning of your meals.

This is a personal step. We all have different tastes and preferences. You have to be able to eat what you like. Eating food that satisfies you without thinking you are leaving half of your life behind because you can't eat ice cream or chips anymore is key. You will be able to eat them from time to time. For the rest of the time, you need to keep the right food available.

Most people think that what's important is the amount of what they eat, which translates into how many calories they are taking in. Include exercise into the equation, and voilà, they have all they need.

The equation for gaining or losing weight as the number of calories in (how much you eat) versus the number of calories out (how much you expend) is quite true, but how and when you consume those calories are also important. These factors are difficult to add to the equation, but their impact is important to the outcome. That's why you need to learn how and when to eat.

In this step, you will learn why it is important to have each of your full meals—breakfast, lunch, and dinner—and two snacks, and how to get organized.

Basic Components of Each Meal

I will ask you to have food from every nutrient group in each meal: carbohydrates, proteins, and fats (except for dinner). The reason is that to accomplish the objective you are interested in here—weight management—you need each component in the meal equilibrium:

> *Carbohydrates* give you the energy to perform your daily activities.

> *Protein,* the building block of muscle, helps you reduce the absorption of sugars and bad fats and provides you with durable energy.

> *Good fats* help you feel satisfied so you stop eating and feel full longer.

> *Fruits, vegetables, and dairy* give you most of the vitamins, minerals, and calcium necessary to be healthy.

Obviously, in each group there are different nutrients with specific benefits, but we are not covering this aspect here.

Although you are going to learn more in future steps, I have listed a few examples of the **most recommended** foods in each general nutrient group:

> **Carbohydrates**: bread, rice, pasta, quinoa, couscous, grains, beans

> **Protein**: egg, cheese, ham, beef, chicken, fish, prosciutto, salami, tofu, beans, nuts. When choosing any of the processed meats, try to use an organic brand or at least one free of nitrites and nitrates.

> **Good fats**: olive oil, avocados, nuts, fatty fish (tuna, salmon, swordfish)

› **Fruit**: all fruits are important, but you should prioritize those lowest in sugar, such as berries, apples, pears, and oranges.

› **Vegetables**: as with fruit, vegetables are all are important and necessary, but avoid those higher in sugars like potatoes, sweet potatoes, and carrots.

› **Dairy:** milk, plain yogurt, light cheese, or kefir (a fermented drink made from milk)

Fermented Foods

An adequate balance of the right bacteria in our body helps with weight management. One of the best ways to get them is by eating fermented food.

And the **less recommended** (and therefore those to avoid):

› **Sugars**, which are a type of carbohydrate: table sugars, candy, jellies, chocolate bars, sugary drinks, juices, cookies, cakes, high fructose corn syrup. You'll also find a list of other names for sugar in Appendix D.

› **Bad fats**: cholesterol from meats (trim as much fat as you can from the meat) and full-fat dairy, trans fats from cookies, crackers, and other processed bakery items, and highly processed foods like stir fries and any sauce you get in many fast food restaurants or in the precooked section of the grocery store

Breakfast Is Your Ally

I am sure you have heard about the importance of breakfast hundreds of times, and I am also sure most of you have never taken it into real consideration.

Breakfast is the boost for your day. It is your start flag. Not only does breakfast give you energy after a whole night on an empty stomach, but it also sets the tone for your metabolism for the rest of the day. If you don't feed your body after a night of fasting, your metabolism will be low, and your body will try to consume as few calories as possible to avoid using scarce resources. A slow metabolism will run low for three, four, five, even six hours, or until you properly feed your body (until lunch). Those are hours your body could use to burn energy.

Many people think that because they didn't ingest food, they saved those calories. This is true, but the results are not as direct and simple as that. After twelve to sixteen hours of fasting, your metabolism goes haywire. By the time you sit down to a meal, you are starving so you eat more than you should. By then, your body craves so much energy that it is going to grab to whatever enters your stomach.

After your overnight fast, your body uses all ingredients to the very last drop, and this is a super-efficient process. And if by any chance there is something left that is not needed right away, it will be stored as fat as soon as possible. If your first food after such a long fasting period is one of those extra-sugary snacks, the insulin boost will make that absorption process still quicker and more effective. Then blood sugar levels will drop drastically, and you will feel the food craving right away. After that, your metabolism will turn to a standby mode of low burning until you have food again.

In contrast, if you eat an appropriate breakfast as soon as you get up, your body will react as it should. During sleeping hours, your metabolism is naturally slow and doesn't need calories. In fact, it works best on a semi-empty stomach. If you then provide the required energy by eating an appropriate breakfast, not only does your metabolism not overreact with an insulin peak, but you'll be providing it with enough energy to avoid running low in a few hours. Bear in mind you are usually most active in the morning, so unless you had a good breakfast, you require a snack before the established time for the next meal, which is usually three or four hours later.

You may have heard about a "new" trend that intermittent fasting helps weight loss, and therefore skipping breakfast is good. I respect this way of thinking as long as your last meal was before 6:00 or 7:00 p.m. (remember, with no carbs at night) to help your weight-loss-management-friendly hormones work properly at night, *and* you don't have a brain-demanding activity in the morning. Your brain needs a *lot* of energy, so you won't be performing well unless you feed that demanding organ. Because of my background in biological science, I personally favor having breakfast because it benefits both your metabolism and your weight management goals. Having said that, if you absolutely hate the idea of having breakfast, and you have tried several times and it doesn't work for you, you'll have to skip this part and work harder in the other aspects of the 32 Mondays Weight Management Program.

So let's take breakfast seriously. You need a low-sugar breakfast, please. No more extra-sugary cereals, pancakes, muffins, and cookies. You can have those from time to time, on that weekend when you have extra time with the family or your partner, or you're alone and want a special breakfast. Once you get used to other types of breakfast, believe me, you won't be missing or craving the sugary ones.

Now, let's discuss what you should be eating for breakfast.

› **Whole-grain carbohydrates & fruits**: bread, rice, pasta, quinoa, couscous, sugar-free oatmeal, sweet potato, and carrots; low-sugar fruit like berries, apple, pears, or oranges. Note: fruit contains a lot of sugar. If you like having fruit in the morning you should consider it as your source of carbohydrate.

› **Protein**: egg, cheese, ham, meat, prosciutto, tofu, nuts, fish

› **Vegetables**: anything you feel like having except for potato, sweet potato, or carrots

› **Dairy**: milk, plain and unsweetened yogurt, kefir, or light cheese

If having all nutrient groups sounds like too much, eat small portions of each group or leave the fruit for lunch or dinner (it fills you without providing enough long-term energy anyway) and the dairy for your snack.

If you like having coffee or tea in the morning, avoid adding sugar. Remember, it is just a matter of changing your taste and your habits. The same goes for yogurt or kefir; try step-by-step to reduce the amount of sugar you add, or maybe use fresh fruit to sweeten them naturally. Commercial fruit and sweetened yogurts and kefirs have too much added sugar, which is totally unnecessary (sweetened or fruit yogurt contains at least 19 grams of sugar per serving compared to 6 to 8 grams in plain yogurt). It is okay to have them from time to time, but not daily.

Dissecting the "Perfect" American Breakfast

Okay, I recognize the great contribution of the "Big American Breakfast" to humanity, and I consider it quite a balanced breakfast. You simply need to adapt it for our purposes here: weight management and a healthy diet.

So if you are thinking fried eggs with bacon, a bagel, and orange juice make the perfect combination, I am sorry to tell you, they do not. While the general approach is good, the specifics are not.

Eggs are a perfect breakfast staple because they contain protein and are not too high in calories—depending on how you prepare them. Forget about fried eggs: those contain an enormous quantity of bad fats and calories, which you don't need. Instead, sauté the same egg. This means using a quality frying pan with a little bit of oil. If you are in a hotel or a restaurant, go easy on omelets and scrambled eggs. You don't realize it because you are used to them, but they are sometimes cooked with lots of oil. Instead, have a hard- or soft-boiled egg. Again, you can cook your omelets and scrambled eggs at home using a tiny quantity of olive oil. Finally, try not to have too many of them. Although eggs are healthy if cooked right , they can be a problem if you have high cholesterol levels. Therefore, eat no more than one a day.

Bacon has an enormous amount of fat. The meat part of the bacon is fine, but the fatty part adds calories with no benefit. When you are at home and you really crave bacon, always remove all fat before cooking it. I know you are removing half of the bacon but think of that fat added to your tummy or butt, or worse, around your liver! You can always go for turkey bacon, which has much less fat. If you are in a hotel or restaurant and you really can't leave without that piece of bacon, always order it well cooked, which means at least part of the fat has been left in the pan. Bacon gives you quite a lot of protein, so it is not that bad as long as you don't have it every day *and* you remove as much fat as possible. Or, try grilling it to get rid of all the fat.

Bagels have a gummy and plastic texture. Any kind of bread with that texture has plenty of ingredients added to make it like that. These include artificial additives that have no health benefits and modified fats for texture. Do not eat these types of bread, as they hide too many additives and unhealthy fats that unnecessarily add too many extra calories to your daily diet. The truth is that nowadays it is difficult to find prepackaged breads that don't have added fats and sugars. I suggest you get baked breads from a bakery or the bakery section of your grocery store. Check the ingredients: although some contain sunflower oil and canola oil (or similar), they don't contain trans fats. The best option is to find breads with no oil or fat and no sugar or honey added, but they are not easy to find unless you buy organic bread (and even then, not always). And please, always go for whole grains and whole wheat; you'll learn why in Step 8. If you are at a hotel buffet or a restaurant, look for hard (not gummy) whole-wheat or whole-grain bread. If those aren't available, at least choose a whole-grain bread or bagel, and eat only half of the portion size. Better yet, grab some granola (usually sweet but at least packed with fiber), nuts, or even fruit. Note: some granola can be packed with a lot of sugar and unhealthy fats, so make sure you have as little as possible.

Orange juice contains plenty of vitamins and minerals. But remember: fruit juices contain a high amount of sugar. When you have juice for breakfast, you are filling your stomach with liquid, and you might not have enough room for proper and filling food to last until lunchtime. You are probably also having coffee or tea, so you feel full easily. Instead of juice, have some small pieces of whole, fresh fruit with its associated fiber. If you absolutely can't live without orange juice in the morning, make sure it doesn't contain added sugar, and have it with pulp if possible. Be aware that hotel buffets usually serve juices with added sugar.

Hash browns, and potatoes in general, have a high glycemic index. Eat them occasionally and try to have them only at home, cooking them with a very small amount of olive oil in a good frying pan.

Sugary cereals should disappear from your diet—and from your children's diets, too! They are packed with unnecessary sugars (or honey, corn syrup, etc.), and they are usually not whole-grain cereals. However, if you go to the organic or "natural foods" department of your grocery store, you will find whole-grain, plain cereals made with rice, corn, and other grains, with no added sugars or any other artificial ingredients. (See my suggested shopping list in Appendix E for suggestions.) If you add them to plain yogurt with some fruit and maybe some granola, you have a perfect bowl of cereal. The kids will love the blueberries and pineapple or kiwi as much as they love the sweet cereal. Believe me, kids are smart, and they recognize good and healthy food when you re-educate them!

Cookies, buns, rolls, coffee cakes, muffins: forget about all of them. They are packed with sugar and fats, most of them with really bad fats. They'll make you full quickly because of the fats, not allowing enough room for some healthy food, but the sugar in them burns too quickly to leave you satisfied for the three to four hours until your next meal. Remember: the high-sugar content generates an undesirable, high-insulin response that make you crave more sugar.

Lunch

You still need quite a lot of energy to make it through the rest of your busy day—and you'll get that with a nutritious lunch. Lunch should be a duplication of your breakfast (protein, carbohydrate, fruit and/or dairy), but will include those foods that most of us would never be able to eat in the morning, like meat, fish, and pasta. So instead of a piece of bread with cheese and ham, have a plate of whole-grain pasta with meatballs (low in fat and organic if possible). You usually don't have time to eat too much, so you need to eat a meal packed with lots of protein in a small serving.

There is nothing healthier and more weight management-friendly than eating your own homemade lunch. It doesn't always need to be a full-cooked meal if you don't have time to cook or don't have enough leftovers. You can put together a pretty decent meal from the local deli with some ham or turkey (organic if possible), low-fat cheese, whole-wheat bread, fruit, and low-fat, unsweetened yogurt, for example.

Let's say you don't have your own cooked or prepared lunch and you need to go out. Try to find a nice salad with some protein like chicken, meat, egg, tuna, beans, or quinoa, or add some nuts as a source of protein to give you enough long-lasting energy to get through the rest of the day. Avoid dressings that are packed with fat and/or sugars; instead use vinegar, olive oil, and lemon juice.

Most of us are not used to having our main meal at lunch instead of dinner, but it is not too difficult to change. In fact, once you give it a try, you will see that you're able to handle the rest of your day much better. You will have more energy, fewer cravings, better concentration, and more stable moods. It is common sense to have a main meal in the middle of the day rather than when you have almost ended your daily activities.

If you don't have access to a microwave to warm your food at lunch, you can try one of those containers that keeps food warm for four to five hours (the same way children do for school). A thermos with soup is another good option. Or you can always have a salad packed with nuts for energy and chicken, meat, or cheese for protein.

Here's what you should be eating for lunch:

> **Whole-grain carbohydrates**: bread, rice, pasta, quinoa, couscous, grains, beans, or starchy vegetables

> **Protein**: eggs, cheese, ham, beef, fish, chicken, prosciutto, salami, tofu, beans, nuts. Remember to get organic processed meat, or at least meat that is nitrite- and nitrate-free.

> **Fruit**: choose low-sugar fruits like berries, apples, pears, or oranges.

> **Vegetables**: some vegetables or a small salad.

> **Dairy**: milk, plain and unsweetened yogurt, kefir, or light cheese

> **Good fats**: olive oil, avocados, nuts, fatty fish (tuna, salmon, swordfish)

Dinner

Now that you have had the bulk of your food for lunch and probably a snack between lunch and dinner (you'll learn about snacking in the next step), you won't arrive at your dinner table as a wild, starving creature, and you can use some sense to plan dinner. You don't need the calories anymore because you will be going to sleep in a few hours, and you need your stomach to be as empty as possible to let your night hormones work properly. In Principle 9, you learned how hormones work in favor of your weight management at night while you sleep. But even if you don't eat a large, high-calorie meal, you still need plenty of vitamins and minerals. Therefore, your dinner should always include:

> › **Protein**: fish, eggs, tofu, ham, cheese, which are all low in calories and easy to digest.

> › **Fruit**: berries, apples, pears, oranges.

> › **Vegetables**: any kind, raw or cooked, except potatoes, sweet potatoes and carrots, which should only be eaten occasionally.

> › **Dairy**: milk, plain and unsweetened yogurt, kefir, or light cheese.

> › **Good fats**: nuts, avocado, olive oil.

These foods are packed with vitamins and minerals, are low in calories and carbohydrates, and are easily digested. By sticking to these foods for your dinner, you will go to sleep without feeling hungry but with your stomach empty enough to sleep well and enjoy the maximum benefit of night hormones.

If you have followed the Menu Plan and have eaten healthy food in the suggested proportions during the day, this is when you could have your small treat, like a piece of chocolate (pure if possible, or as high a percentage of cocoa as possible), a cookie (trans-fat free and whole-wheat or whole-grain if possible), or one of the other treats we've mentioned earlier. The idea of having a treat after dinner can help you behave during the day and at dinner and will help you make the right choices when organizing your meals and snacks.

Snacks

I have mentioned snacks in several steps and in the principles. A snack at the right time allows you to get to the next complete meal in equilibrium so you won't jump desperately into the food. In fact, snacking is such an important subject that I've devoted the next step to covering all the important information you'll need.

Organizing Meals: Efficiency and Planning

I am completely aware of how much I am asking of you when I say you need a proper breakfast, lunch, dinner, and snacks! Well, there are two words that can lead you to succeed: **efficiency and planning**.

I am giving you enough information in this step that you will be able to organize the right number of meals with the right composition. Not only you are going to lose weight without being hungry, but you will lose weight because you are already starting to eat the right way to lose weight.

According to Merriam-Webster.com, the definition of **efficiency** is "The ability to do something or produce something without wasting materials, time, or energy."

You began this Program five weeks ago. You have learned to manage the grocery store so you will always have necessary ingredients at home. You have also learned how important it is to prepare your own meals and how to find time to cook and how to do so as efficiently as possible.

Well, to be as efficient as possible in preparing your meals, you need **planning**. I learned this saying from my young daughter: "Failing to plan is planning for failure," and I believe it applies to weight loss and healthy living, too.

Always plan ahead for meals and lunches that are easy to bring to the office, to school, or to warm up and eat at home. When you plan your meals ahead of time, you are taking away one responsibility and therefore leaving one less thing you have to think about during the day. You need to know what you are preparing to be able to have the ingredients and set aside the necessary time to prepare or cook them. But where should you start?

I suggest you make a list of meals that you already know how to prepare. Write the recipe on a card, and add other cards with variations of those same meals, and make a new card for each new meal you learn to prepare; the more you have, the more varied your meal plans will be.

Use those cards to prepare your weekly meal plan and to know which ingredients you will need to put on your grocery list for all three daily meals and snacks.

Remember to use the proposed shopping list in Appendix E and the meal plan in Appendix F.

Tip: Always plan your menus in the morning, after a good night's sleep and a healthy breakfast, when your willpower is in full supply and you are still relaxed and not hungry. You'll be able to make better choices when planning your menus.

As you learned in Principle 5, stock your fridge and cabinets with ingredients you'll need to fix quick but nourishing meals. You can always freeze some cooked leftovers to have at least one or two meals available for emergencies. Use dinner leftovers from a couple of days ago for lunch.

Again, if your dinnertime is really early, you should switch your afternoon snack for your after-dinner snack at night or save part of the afternoon snack and part of dinner to eat as a night snack. But remember, no food within two hours of going to bed.

Eating Out

Restaurants, and especially all-you-can-eat buffets, can be a minefield for anyone who is concerned about healthy eating. While you certainly have more control over your choices when you prepare your own meals, there are occasions when that just isn't an option. At those times, you'll need to remember a few tricks to make sure you stay on the 32 Mondays Weight Management Program.

Business Meals

It is a total misconception that a meal has to be rich and filling to be considered a good meal. In fact, the trendy *nouvelle cuisine* is based on frugal plates and meals, and the trendiest meals are now Mediterranean, which is known for mild and healthy ingredients. Being healthy is "in"! Having a 22-ounce steak with a lot of fries is less trendy than having a light salad with olive oil and vinegar and grilled fish.

You can use this to your advantage during a business lunch or dinner. Your associate's perception will be: This person is healthy, dynamic, and under control. He or she eats light and concentrates on business. Food is secondary; business is important.

With this in mind, when having business meals, apply the same concepts for the everyday lunch with the only exception that you may be eating in a nicer restaurant. There are always light salads and soups (avoid creamy soups) to choose from. Other options are any grilled meat or fish prepared without added butter; remember that most restaurants add butter to grilled food for flavor. Another good option is brown rice or whole-wheat pasta without too much sauce. Sauces are usually what can change a healthy, light meal into a heavy, high-calorie one. Remember to ask the waitstaff for lower-calorie, lower-fat options that might be available but not on the menu. If appropriate, go ahead with some wine, but remember not to overdo it; you want to avoid the powerful feeling that makes you go for more food and the extra and unnecessary calories. Feel like having dessert? Remember, this is a business meal where you are working, so try not to eat an excessive dessert that might leave you feeling full and slow. Save some carbs from your meal and order a small ice cream, flan, or crème brûlée, something with proteins and not just sugars.

Vacations, Celebrations, and Other Special Occasions

You behave most of the time, eating light and healthy, and from time to time you want to be able to treat yourself. Enjoy a good treat when it's time to celebrate a special occasion. Just remember, at the same time you have been changing your eating habits, you have also changed your digestive system. If you have been avoiding fried food, creamy sauces and soups, and fatty meats for a while, you will probably now have trouble digesting your meal if you have those in excess. You will end up ingesting lots of calories and not enjoying the experience while feeling sick and tired. Think carefully about your choice at the restaurant. Let's say you really feel like having a nice steak, a saucy pasta or rice, or a fried choice. Eat only salad with it, and avoid creamy soups or seasonings. Go for a light dessert. Enjoy a cocktail or a glass of beer or wine, but only one. If what you are really looking forward to is dessert, eat a light meal, like a salad or a light soup and a grilled fish or meat, and then dip into your chocolate cake. You have to think carefully about your options and choose wisely so you'll enjoy the special occasion and not end up feeling stuffed and tired.

All-You-Can-Eat Buffets

It is quite easy to overeat at a buffet unless you have a plan. Before you begin selecting food, first have a look at the entire buffet and decide what you are going to eat and then stay with your selection.

If you are having lunch (dinner shouldn't have the carbs but the concept applies!) and whole-wheat pasta is what is really tempting you, make that your choice for your main course and then just choose a medium fruit or a yogurt for dessert. If it is the cake or ice cream or other dessert that is really calling you, go with just a big salad with some cheese and nuts or a small salad and a small piece of meat, fish, or egg, and then go for the dessert. In any case, forget about bread. You are probably going to eat more than the recommended portion sizes, so forget any additional food. Take no more than three trips: one for the salad/soup, one for the main course, and one for dessert.

If you are having breakfast at the buffet, the initial survey of the buffet still applies so you can see all the options and decide on the best one. Breakfast buffets are often packed with unhealthy muffins and other sweets. Just forget about them. The bread is also usually highly processed and there may be no whole-wheat bread, but if you find a good option you can have toast with cream cheese or eggs. Another good option is a plain yogurt with some nuts and/or muesli.

Restaurant Tips

Although you don't know exactly how food is prepared in a restaurant, and most of the time it is with too much fat, if you eat out from time to time, here are a few tips for enjoying a healthy, satisfying meal without feeling deprived:

› Food is only a small part of any celebration or outing. Try to focus on the social part of the event to avoid giving too much importance to food.

› Don't arrive hungry to the restaurant. It is difficult to make the right choices when you feel hungry. Plan a snack beforehand according to the time of the meal.

› Plan in advance by checking the menu online and making the right choices at home when you are calm and not hungry. Decide if you are going for a heavier meal and no dessert, or a light meal with a rich dessert. If you can't access the menu online, take your time studying the menu once at the restaurant; decide on your order before you are distracted by a conversation or by the waiter asking for drinks.

› Avoid any alcoholic drinks before ordering the food. They make you feel hungrier, and you will end up eating and drinking more. When the waiter takes drink orders, request just plain water. Wait to order your drink until your meal is served. In the meantime, drink your water to fill up and trick your stomach a bit so you can avoid the bread and butter.

› Refuse bread when it comes—if you can—or if not, place it far away from you. It is usually white, sticky bread packed with empty calories that will make you feel even hungrier after the insulin peak. If you really want to have bread with your meal, order whole-grain bread with no butter.

› Start with a salad or light soup to fill you up.

›   Restaurant portions are out of control! Get smaller portions: split an entrée with somebody; order an appetizer or side as an entrée; or ask to wrap up part of your meal before you even start to eat. Try to split desserts as they also tend to be huge.

›   If you are ordering a piece of meat, look for cuts with less fat. If you don't know, ask the waiter.

›   Choose healthy sides: vegetables with no butter or salad are the best choices.

›   Restaurant dressings and sauces are heavy; avoid them as much as possible, or order dressings and sauces on the side and use only a small portion.

›   Avoid fried food, too much cheese, and creamy sauces and soups.

›   Ask for details about how the entrée is actually prepared.

›   Ask for special orders when there is nothing that suits you, or make sure you eat a small portion.

›   Avoid foods that you suspect might contain too much monosodium glutamate (MSG). Although it might be used in almost any pre-pared food, it is most common in Asian food, sauces, snack foods, and salad dressings.

›   And remember, every bite counts!

SUGGESTED TIME FRAME

I have allowed two weeks to reorganize what you eat and when you eat your meals, but some of you might need more than two weeks to master this step. That is perfectly all right. Just keep going with the next steps of the Program at the same time that you keep working on this one, and you will eventually master it.

I suggest you set objectives for yourself according to how difficult you view the goal. For example, if you have always avoided breakfast, you might need more than one week to get into the routine of having breakfast. Or you might be okay with breakfast but need two weeks to start eating lunch properly and two more to change dinner menus and reduce the amount of rich food and extra calories you eat at night. It is up to your specific needs and background for how much time you take, but before starting, set a time line and follow it. For most people it should take about two weeks to master the step, so use that timing as your goal.

TAKE 5

› **Learn**: Understand why the number, organization, and composition of meals is important.

› **Goal**: Follow the proposed meals with the right composition.

› **Plan**: Use the morning for planning your meals.

› **Monitor**: Check your food journal.

› **Reward**: Treat yourself with fancy menu planner.

KEY POINTS

› Eat breakfast for energy: carbohydrate, protein, and maybe fruit or dairy.

› Eat lunch for energy: carbohydrate, protein, healthy fat, and fruit or dairy.

› Eat a light dinner: non-starchy vegetables, easy-to-digest protein, fruit or dairy.

› Allow three to four hours between meals.

› Don't consume any food two hours before bed.

› Use a card system to register current meals and variations, and add new cards as you learn to prepare new menu items.

› Follow a shopping list to have all the necessary ingredients.

› Follow the menu template found in Step 1.

STEP 5
SNACKING

SUGGESTED TIME FRAME: 2 WEEKS

Snacking is tricky. On one hand, you can't be eating all day, and you need to wait three or four hours between meals. On the other, you don't want to wait more than three to four hours or you'll get too hungry and overeat, and your metabolism will go crazy assimilating all that food. Therefore, ideally you should eat a snack between your main meals so you can maintain the no-more/no-less rule of three to four hours between meals.

Let's see how can you accomplish this.

In Step 4, you learned you need to rest three to four hours between meals to let your metabolism do its work, but no more than that to avoid cravings that will lead you to overeat or to eat inappropriate foods. Also, if you wait longer to eat, your metabolism becomes super efficient, using the calories you eat after five to eight hours since your last meal. It is okay for your body to efficiently absorb vitamins, minerals, and other nutrients, but in terms of calories (energy), you want some of them wasted so you need more available, and your body also gets into a burning mode so you get energy from stored fat. When your system is "too hungry" for calories, it will use all of them.

Another good reason to follow the three-to-four-hour rule is the demonstrated link between low glucose levels and lack of self-control. If you maintain stable glucose levels during the day, you will be able to make better choices.

Blood Glucose

Here you can see another cycle. Your brain needs glucose to make the right decisions. If you haven't eaten in three to four hours, your glucose levels are low. Therefore your self-control runs low, too, resulting in poor food choices while your brain keeps asking for more glucose, which causes more glucose disequilibrium.

You have met the enemy, and you know it! After sugary drinks, snacking is your worst enemy because sugary and high-carb snacks will destabilize your blood glucose equilibrium. These include not only cookies, muffins, and candy bars, but also chips, pretzels, crackers, Frappuccino and similar iced beverages, ice cream, and even fruit, protein bars, and nuts which are considered "healthy" snacks.

To refresh your memory, let's look again at insulin. Every time you snack, no matter how tiny or how healthy your snack is, you send messages to your body that food is available, so all the metabolic mechanisms get ready to act. If this was a tiny snack, insulin was there doing its job, but it was required only for a small action. Every other mechanism (insulin receptors and all the hormones related to glucose regulation, like leptin and ghrelin) was on alert but didn't have too much to do, so they went back to their routines. If you keep doing this day after day, several times a day, guess what? You are going to end up being tired—very tired. You are constantly activating whole mechanisms with no real necessity. That brings uncertainty and misinterpretation to your body's systems. In the end, it will decrease the effectiveness of your regulatory systems to maintain your body's equilibrium. Your body has mechanisms in place to indicate when you have had enough food, when to stop eating, and when to burn more calories. Those mechanisms are your weight management team. When you subject your body to a constant ingestion of food and drinks at any time, you are asking your weight management team to be constantly alert, and in the end, these systems get tired and confused.

They lose the ability to be precise in their work. They don't send the right signals. In the end: chaos!

How Snacking Affects Your Body

If you wait three to four hours between meals, your weight management team is fully relaxed, and it knows exactly what to do, which is good. But if that snack is a high-sugar snack, it will be absorbed quickly by the hormone insulin. There won't be any glucose left so the mechanisms to make you hungry will be activated to make you eat and recover your blood sugar levels. You will then want to eat another snack before the three- to four-hour break is over, and you will enter in a cycle of constantly having high and lows in glucose levels, which will make you hungry, and you will end up eating most of the time.

However, if you not only wait three to four hours between meals, but also have a low-sugar snack that is high in fiber and protein and includes some good fat, things will be different. Your weight management team, which will be rested and efficient after a three- to four-hour break, will need more time to process this snack due to its composition (low in sugar and high in fiber and protein). Your body has no need to rush to lower the levels of sugar in the bloodstream, so the system can take the required time to do a proper job. Protein and fiber (vegetables, fruits, and whole-grain cereals like whole-wheat pasta, bulgur, quinoa, brown rice, and whole-grain bread) take longer to process. It is a much more difficult process than with simple sugars. If immediate energy is required, those complex nutrients must be transformed into simple ones, ready for use, which takes time and energy—in fact, you'll already be spending energy by making them available to your body. Also, because these complex nutrients take longer to digest, you will feel full for a longer period. You will be perfectly able to wait three or four hours until your next meal, allowing your weight management team to recover peacefully.

In addition, enjoying a healthy snack three to four hours after a meal will help you avoid being extra hungry when you get to the next meal so you don't overeat. Instead, your system will make good use of your snacks and meals in a relaxed manner, using the last micro calorie of the ingested food to make it available to your organs. Your body uses what is needed and consumes some energy during the process. On the other hand, when your calories are restricted, your body learns how to burn as few calories as possible by lowering your metabolism. Your body will then expend as few calories as possible during your daily routine. When you put your body into starvation mode, it economizes and slows your metabolism, storing energy and absorbing as much as possible of any little intake of energy. Your body doesn't differentiate between real famine or dieting; everything is just a cut in calorie intake, so your body generates a response by saving as much as possible.

The time for a snack is often not a convenient one. It catches us in the office, attending meetings, on the train, in the car, dropping kids off at their activities, and a host of other inopportune times. You need to be extra cautious about snacking to avoid getting caught in one of those bad craving moments when you eat whatever you have close at hand. When you feel hungry someplace where you don't have anything healthy on hand, you'll end up eating *anything* you can find. Those are usually extra calories you don't even recognize. If you have already started your food diary (which you should have), you can look back and check how many snacks you have had in a week that you haven't planned for.

Always carry easy and convenient snacks: an apple, some cheese with whole-wheat crackers, a bunch of nuts, plain Greek yogurt. Try to avoid sugary cereal bars, juices, or sugary yogurt, and eat those only if accompanied by whole grains, some protein, and/or some good fat to reduce the insulin peak.

Nighttime Snacking

Given our traditional organization of meals, nighttime is the most popular time for snacking. You have dinner early, and you still have a few hours before going to sleep. This is the time most of us finally relax after a long day at work and/or with the kids. You finally sit down. Relax. Get a book. Turn on the TV. Talk to your friend, your partner and… eat! Those are also times you associate with pleasure, and that makes you think you are deriving pleasure just from the food, not from the relaxing time or the pleasant company.

Again, it is the food and beverage industry, hand in hand with the marketing industry, that has developed a way to make us associate good times, enjoyment, pleasure, and happiness with a specific food or drink. Think about all those commercials that market chocolates, ice creams, ranch sauces, fried chicken, chips, and other snack foods.

You need to break the link between eating and those other pleasurable activities. You don't have to eat every time you are in one of those situations, and it is not food that is making you enjoy the moment—it is the activity!

To avoid nighttime snacking, eat your dinner a little bit later. Another strategy is to brush your teeth two hours before going to bed. You will have to choose between the impulse of eating a snack and the laziness of having to brush your teeth again!

If you are following my advice of having your largest meal at lunchtime, and you had a snack three to four hours after your lunch, you should be able to delay your dinnertime. If there is no way that those changes will work for you, go ahead with a snack, but do not eat between two and three hours before bedtime, and avoid carbohydrates. Snacks that contain carbohydrates activate a sugar response that doesn't work well with ghrelin and growth factor hormone release (which you'll learn about in Step 13). Instead, go for what I call perfect, allied snacks.

Perfect, Allied Snacks

Perfect, allied snacks are snacks that are easy to carry everywhere you might need them and are low in sugar and low on the glycemic index. A good example is a serving of nuts—toasted, not fried—and no sugar, honey, or chocolate coverings. Depending on the size of the nut, one serving is between ten and twenty nuts, which is around 165 to 185 calories. Also, you should try to control your salt intake, so choose unsalted snacks.

One thing about nuts, though: they are so yummy and easy to eat that it is difficult to stop and to know when enough is enough. Try to get a prepackaged bag of nuts or pack your own following the recommended serving sizes. Don't carry more than one serving with you.

Here is a list of a one-serving size of other perfect, allied snacks:

> › 1 slice (equal to the size of your thumb) of cheese

> › 1 slice of whole-grain bread

> › 1 medium apple

> › 1 medium pear

> › 1 cup carrots or celery

> › ½ cup hummus

> › ½ avocado

> › 2 slices of ham

> › 1 egg

For a bit of variety, you can combine ½ serving of one snack with ½ serving of another. If you are having carbohydrates, try to combine them with protein or fat. All of the above snacks are around 150 to 200 calories.

Overcome Your Desire for Sugar

I know, you *feel* that eating that cookie—or that candy bar or sugary drink—in the middle of your horrible morning or afternoon saves your life… but it doesn't! That euphoria you feel after your sugary snack is just the sugar peak! As soon as the insulin team removes it, you feel tired and irritable: you have mobilized a big team just for a sugary snack, and now you not only feel as miserable as you were before you ate the snack, but you are *hungry* again because the insulin has removed *all* sugar!

If inappropriate snacks are some of your worst enemies, try to avoid them. Don't have them at home, don't go to the candy jar at work, and don't carry any in your pockets. When you are facing the temptation, just think how bad they will make your body feel afterward, and think about your treat after lunch or dinner. If it is really time for a snack—three to four hours since your last meal—go for a healthy one. And remember, always have a healthy snack handy!

SUGGESTED TIME FRAME

You have two weeks to break the habit of eating snacks all day long and not having proper meals. By now you should have mastered Step 4, where you learned about the number and organization of your daily meals. If you are already eating those healthy and fulfilling meals, you just need to add your healthy snack or snacks between meals.

You might want to use one week to manage the number of snacks and the other week to learn about your healthy snacks, or use both weeks to learn both things at the same time. It is up to you!

TAKE 5

› **Learn**: Understand why the wrong snacks are bad and the good ones at the right time are important.

› **Goal**: Follow the proposed number of recommended snacks.

› **Plan**: Plan and prepare your snacks in the morning with the day's schedule in mind.

› **Monitor**: Use your food journal.

› **Reward**: Treat yourself to a nice watch to help you remember the hours between meals and snacks.

KEY POINTS

› You need three to four hours between meals to let your body do its work in a relaxed and effective manner.

› Eating more than three to four hours after the last meal activates your insulin response and doesn't allow a proper rest for optimum functioning.

> If you don't eat within three to four hours of your last meal, your metabolism activates a high hunger response, resulting in an excessive response to save energy.

> Sugary snacks activate a high insulin response and make you crave more sugar soon afterward.

> Don't associate a snack with an activity. You get pleasure from the movie, TV, book, or friend, not from the popcorn, chips, candy bar, or ice cream.

> Healthy snacks are those low in sugars that contain proteins and some healthy fats.

> Choose a healthy snack from the perfect, allied snacks suggested.

> Always have your healthy snacks on hand and for emergencies.

> Don't eat any snacks two hours before bedtime.

STEP 6
FATS

SUGGESTED TIME FRAME: 4 WEEKS

Of all the bad guys starring in our show, this is the one with the worst press. Fat was the first thing blamed when more and more people started gaining weight a few decades ago. Fat was blamed as the ultimate culprit for the changes in our body shape. Today, we know diets low in fat prevent you from losing weight, and some fats may even help you to lose weight.

After low-fat diets reduced fat to a minimum, carbohydrates became the enemy, then it was meat, then fruit, then back to fat, then protein mixed with carbohydrates.

Well, either we don't have a clue about what is going on, or the truth is we can't blame only one bad guy. The reality is there is never one single factor responsible for something. A bad guy cannot succeed unless he has accomplices, or the right weapons, or has someone on the inside, or because of the good guys arriving late.

It is true that in general, we haven't had a clue for many years. Science changes quickly, so what we might see now as a certainty might not be so in a few months or years. The scientific community is continually researching, and more and better research tools are available each year. So, it is not that strange that "absolutes" change quickly, and we need to view these "truths" with some perspective. To me, there is never one absolute truth, and the main concept in this complex problem is *equilibrium.*

In terms of fat, it is difficult to get to *equilibrium* in your diet—not because you eat too much direct fat, but because of the hidden fats in the processed food you eat. If you don't know what you are eating, how can you ever reach an equilibrium in your diet?

Good versus Bad Fats

Let's talk about the paradigm of the French people, which I mentioned in Step 1. The French eat high amounts of butter and cheese, which are rich in fat and cholesterol, and they don't become especially overweight and don't even have a higher cholesterol level than other groups. The reason is not the fat they eat per se, but the fat they don't eat. Not only do they eat smaller portion sizes than we do, but they also don't eat hidden fat.

French people *love* food. They like to shop for fresh food, cook it, and eat it. It is difficult to find a French person opening the freezer to look for a pre-cooked meal or getting takeout from a fast-food restaurant. Of course, things are changing everywhere, but I bet you it will take longer for the processed-food industry to succeed in France than anywhere else.

The Mediterranean diet has also been closely observed. Although diets in the Mediterranean countries are changing, there are still specific traits to characterize them—fresh fruit and vegetables, olive oil, nuts, and fish. The number of people who are overweight in those countries, although increasing, is still under control. It is not that they don't eat fat, (you'd be amazed how much olive oil is consumed in those countries), but fast food and ready-to-eat meals packed with hidden modified fats are still a minor part of their diets.

I have been showing you our real enemy is not fat per se, but the amount and type of fat that gets into your body that you are not even aware you are eating. Now, let's review the difference between good and bad fats.

We need fat. Some important constituents of our metabolism, including some hormones, are "fat" based because they are generated from fat. But you need the good one.

Good Fats

To make it simple and easy to remember, we'll define good fats as the unprocessed ones, in general unprocessed oils and fats from fruits, vegetables, and fish. Animal fats, other than fish, although not really bad, raise bad cholesterol, which is absolutely necessary for our body, but it becomes harmful when in excess. That means you need to keep a close eye on how much animal fat you are eating.

Bad Fats

Again, to make it simple, consider any fat that has been processed in one way or another a bad fat. It could be in the form of cooked fat (fried food), or fat processed before being used (modified fat, for example, trans fat). Those fats are bad for two reasons: first they are unhealthy for your body, and second, they are hidden in most of the foods you find, so you are not even aware you are overeating them. You can find them in breads, crackers, some cheese spreads, margarine and butter substitutes, cookies, waffles, pancakes, and all sorts of precooked meals.

Modified fats, especially hydrogenated fats, are nowadays the golden ingredient used to improve the taste, palatability (how you feel the food in your mouth), and shelf life of almost all processed foods. They are so common in all foods that it is difficult to avoid them unless you study the labels of almost every food in your house. Sometimes it is practically impossible to avoid them unless you cook the products yourself, as in the case of cookies and almost every cake and muffin.

You have been unconsciously educated to appreciate that feeling of food's soft melting in your mouth. The food manufacturing industry realized that when they added those bad fats to basic meals, we tended to eat more because those bad fats made the product easier to eat. Let's look at the example of bread.

Bread was invented in the Neolithic period, and its evolution in history has been based on ingredient availability. For centuries, and still today in some European countries like France, Spain, Italy, and Greece, bread is more of a dried product, crusty and crumbly.

In the United States, we have been educated to eat soft, sticky bread, so easy to munch that it takes us only a second before we are ready for more, so we end up eating more than we should. Although the base for bread is wheat, water, and raising agents, bad fats have been added to increase softness and palatability. This is the same situation with most flour-based products like cookies and muffins, where fats are added to give us more pleasure when we eat them. (By the way, soft bread also contains significant amounts of sugar.)

The thing is, you can change your tastes. You don't need to be pawns of the food industry. You can go back to eating just "normal" bread, like a French baguette or Italian ciabatta. Enjoy any of those breads with some fresh tomato and a drop of olive oil.

When it comes to processed food, there is not much you can do except be careful reading labels, and using natural and organic brands as much as possible, which tend not to use modified fats and other bad fats. Try to avoid processed food and cook food yourself so you know exactly what you are feeding your body.

Types of Fat and Your Health

As we've discussed in previous sections, there are several types of fats: some good, others not that good, and others bad or really bad. Some of them interfere with the metabolism of cholesterol. For what you are concerned with here, you only need to know that HDL (high-density lipoprotein) is the good cholesterol you want to have because it helps reduce heart disease risk. LDL (low-density lipoprotein) is bad cholesterol you want to avoid because it increases the risk of heart disease and some types of cancer. Triglycerides (metabolized fat) also must be kept under control.

Saturated Fats

Basically, these fats are found in animal products (including beef, poultry, pork, dairy and its sub products like ice cream, butter, and cheese), but there are also some vegetable sources such as tropical oils, including palm oil and palm kernel oil.

They are bad because they raise LDL, but not as bad some others because they also increase HDL.

Saturated fats need to be eaten in moderation. You usually eat more than necessary, so it is important to move to low-fat milk products and trim poultry and meat. Be careful with having too much of those fats. They seem to be directly related with how much belly fat you carry.

Unsaturated Fats

Unsaturated fats are excellent. For good health, the majority of fats you eat should be monounsaturated and polyunsaturated.

Monounsaturated fats, such as extra-virgin olive oil, nuts, avocado, sesame, and peanut oils increase HDL (good) and lower LDL (bad). They protect against heart disease. Some authors and researchers[16] say they help to burn fat, even up to five hours after the meal and help you eat less. They activate the fat metabolism and make you feel full when included in a meal, making you eat less.

Polyunsaturated

Two types of fat make up this category: omega-6 and omega-3 fats, which also need to be in the correct ratio (between 1:1 and 5:1) for optimal health benefits. Right now most Americans have a range of 20-50:1.[17,18,19]

Omega-3 fats are found in salmon, tuna, mackerel, shad, sardines, trout, shark, swordfish, and fish in general. Flaxseeds, walnuts, canola and soy oils, tofu, cauliflower, broccoli, and cabbage also have omega-3.

Omega-3 protects against cardiovascular disease and increases good (HDL) cholesterol. One of the reasons for the health benefits of the Mediterranean diet is the high consumption of fish rich in omega-3. It reduces inflammation and risk of heart attack, and it benefits other conditions. Studies suggest it helps you regulate your weight and helps you burn more fat more efficiently[20,21]. Omega-3s are also associated with mental illness improvement.

This is an excellent fat! You absolutely need it, yet most people never eat enough of it. You need to actively try to have more. If there is no way to increase your consumption of fish to at least twice a week, one of my few supplement recommendations is to take a fish oil (omega-3) supplement. (For more about supplements, see Part III.)

Omega-6 fats are found in walnuts, flaxseeds, pumpkin, and sunflower seeds. Safflower, sesame, and corn oils are also sources of omega-6.

They lower both good (HDL) and bad (LDL) cholesterol. They are good fats when eaten in moderation and in proper proportion with omega-3s.

A word of caution: An excess of omega-6 fats has recently been associated with inflammation and blood vessel damage with subsequent health effects[22].

Keep an eye on your intake of omega-6 fats. Corn is in many foods, so you can easily end up having too much. Eat almonds, walnuts, and pumpkin and sunflower seeds that are also rich in omega-3 and do not have the negative effects of canola, soy, and corn oils, which are highly processed. Many of the latter come from genetically engineered sources.

Industrial Trans Fats

Hydrogenated vegetable fats and shortening are added to many industrial foods like cookies, bread, cereals, crackers, dressings, margarines, popcorn, fried foods, toppings… the list can go on and on. They are also found in most fried foods.

They increase LDL, the bad kind of cholesterol, and lower HDL, the good kind of cholesterol. They also increase inflammation and heart weakening and are associated with many other negative health effects, *including weight gain.*

Be careful when reading labels. Although manufacturers have to list trans fats by law, they only have to list them when the quantity is larger than a certain amount. They are careful to stay under the limit or to suggest a smaller serving size that doesn't reach the reportable minimum threshold that requires listing. So even if you see trans fats as 0 grams, you could be in trouble if you eat two of those small cookies! The serving is so small that the trans fat content falls below the reportable threshold. Always check the list of ingredients to look for words like *partially hydrogenated oil* (usually palm or other vegetable fat) or *shortening*. Another tricky fact is that because trans fats are solids at normal temperatures, you don't recognize the fatty feeling associated with the normal form of what was used: oil. So it is much more difficult for the consumer to recognize these fats. Instead of an oily feeling, you have a delicious texture!

Regarding all fried commercial foods, almost all of them are fried in trans fats because those fats are easier to ship and store in a restaurant.

These are really bad fats. You need to actively avoid them as much as possible.

Practical Tips to Reduce the Amount of Fat and Choose Only the Good Ones

- *Avoid fried food: French fries, chips, chicken nuggets, fried fish, fried nuts… you don't need that extra fat in your body. Eat them only occasionally, once a week or less. Go instead for a baked potato, grilled chicken or fish, and natural nuts.*

- *Avoid precooked meals as much as possible. If you have no choice but to have them, check the labels and go for the brands with less fat and no trans fats.*

- *Avoid industrial cakes, muffins, cookies, and other baked goods. Read the labels carefully to avoid the worst fats (hydrogenated and shortening) and try to go organic as much as possible since those products usually contain healthier ingredients. Cook your own from scratch, or at least use organic mixes as much as possible.*

- *Drink skim milk, yogurt, kefir, and other low-fat dairy products.*

- *Eat low-fat cheese.*

- *Trim all meat and poultry as much as possible and remove the skin before cooking. Try to always choose lean pieces.*

- *Avoid margarine (with hydrogenated oils and fats). Use a bit of butter on your bread, or even better, try olive oil instead.*

- *Cook with less fat (butter or oil). Learn how to use a minimum amount of fat when using the right pans.*

- *Bake, grill, or stir-fry rather than fry.*

- *Avoid candy bars as treats as much as possible because they are packed with bad fats.*

- *Reduce the amount of dressing in your salad, or much better, start to use vinegar and a little bit of olive oil.*

- *Eat fish twice a week, and at least once a week eat salmon, mackerel, or sardines. Eat tuna only once every two weeks because mercury tends to accumulate in the body. Eat wild fish as much as you can to avoid fish raised on dry food. Always look for wild salmon—research suggests it contains more omega-3 than the farm-raised equivalent. Be careful with eating too much shellfish since it filters toxins which in excess can be harmful.*

- *Eat more nuts, but be careful, as it is easy to eat too many. A handful a day as a snack is more than enough.*

- *Eat flaxseed.*

- *Move to olive oil. Look for extra-virgin, cold-pressed olive oil.*

- *Avoid vegetable oils like canola, corn, soy, safflower. They are manufactured using chemical products and/or high tempera-tures and as a consequence include trans fats. Many are also genetically modified (GMO).*

- *Take an omega-3 supplement if you are not eating enough fish.*

SUGGESTED TIME FRAME

I have allowed four weeks for you to master this step. It presents a certain degree of difficulty since you need to learn about different types of fat and where they are present. You also need to continue to read labels, and most important, change your eating and shopping habits, which you should have started doing already.

To begin this step, I suggest you first stop eating fried foods and move to alternative choices. Then replace full-fat for skim-milk products. Trim meats and poultry. Empty your cabinets of all fatty cookies, muffins, and other similar products. Spend one morning or afternoon at the grocery store reading labels of alternative cooked meals like a frozen entrée (for emergencies), cookies and other baked goods (for your treats), and other products you might need in the kitchen (like tomato sauce). This is a research project, so you need to make a list of those products and brands you have identified as suitable replacements for what is less healthy.

Finally, learn how to cook low-fat meals by using a minimum amount of cooking oil and by using the right low-fat products like trimmed meat, low-fat cheese, and organic, low-fat chicken broth. Start moving from different types of vegetable oils to cold-pressed olive oil, the healthiest one.

At the end of four weeks, you'll have mastered this step and will be well on your way to a healthier lifestyle.

TAKE 5

› **Learn**: Understand which are the good and the bad fats.

› **Goal**: Minimize the consumption of bad fats by eating some good fats in each meal.

› **Plan**: Organize your daily menus without bad fats and with some good fats in each meal.

› **Monitor**: Continue to enter your meals in the food journal.

> › **Reward**: Treat yourself to a nice plate, tray, or something similar with a variety of nuts every week.

KEY POINTS

> › Avoid trans fats as much as possible. They are hidden in industrial breads, cakes, cookies, chips, and most processed foods.

> › Read labels to detect trans fats: other names are hydrogenated oils or shortening.

> › Go for organic as much as possible to avoid trans fat.

> › Avoid eating too much corn-based food, which contains excess omega-6.

> › Avoid too much fat from animal sources: fatty meats, chicken, and dairy.

> › Go for lean cuts of meats, remove fat from meat and chicken, remove skin from chicken, and have skim milk and dairy products.

> › Eat more olive oil, avocado, nuts, flaxseed, and fish.

> › Do not remove all fat from your diet. It helps you burn fat and feel full and satisfied after a meal.

> › Take an omega-3 supplement if you are not eating fish at least two to three times per week.

STEP 7
SUGARS

Now that you understand how sugar impacts the insulin response and how that affects your weight loss, and you have also stopped drinking sugary drinks, you are well on your way to achieving your weight management goals.

Some people tend to think that sugars per se are not really "that" bad. They increase tooth decay, of course, but still have half the calories of fat and the same number as protein. I think this is the reason the press hasn't been as bad for sugar as it has for fat. Sugary food is so tasty, so energizing, and has so many ways to eat it that it is difficult to say no to it. Why should you say no when it is lower in calories than fat and much more fun and tastier than protein?

The reality is that sugars *are* bad. They activate a huge response in your body that makes your metabolism stay fully alert, including the huge insulin reaction. They are also so simple to process that they are easily transformed into fat and don't even require much energy to accomplish that. Review the principles of the 32 Mondays Weight Management Program for more details.

Sugar comes in multiple forms, and you might not know all its names. This means you might not recognize other terms for sugar when reading food labels. You'll find a full list of other names for sugar in Appendix D; print the list and keep it in a handy place for when you go shopping. Also, try to read it from time to time and learn the names so you are able to recognize them on labels.

The World Health Organization recommends a maximum of 10 percent of the total energy intake come from sugars, roughly 50 grams or 12 teaspoons of sugar per day[23]; a further reduction to 25 grams a day or 6 teaspoons would provide additional health benefits. The average American is eating more than 30 teaspoons (120 grams) of sugar a day—and much of that is hidden. Those teaspoons are not in your tea, that's for sure, so check for some of them in other processed foods you are eating: all types of sugar including brown and beet, sucrose, cane juice, fructose or fruit juices, galactose, maltose, molasses, and any syrups, including corn, rice, and malt. Please note that brown sugar, often lauded for being healthy, only differs from white sugar in its taste and some added minerals. Therefore, for the purpose of weight management, it should be considered exactly the same as white sugar.

One of the most pressing problems with sugar is that it is present in most foods, especially in the typical snacks you tend to eat. Think about those cookies, energy bars, candies, ice creams, and muffins you like to have for a snack. You have already learned about snacking and how sugary snacks hurt your weight loss.

To make things worse, the food manufacturing industry has also learned a great deal about sugar and the addiction it generates. When sugars are added to most foods, that food ends up being tastier—so much tastier, in fact, that nowadays most processed foods have sugar in their composition—even salad dressing, bread, mayonnaise, beans, and tomato sauce. Even meat foods like sausages contain added sugar.

Please, go back to Part I of this book and refer to **Principle 7: Physical and Psychological Food Addictions**. You will understand much more about sugar and about your metabolic reaction to it, which will help you manage your physical and mental cravings for sugar. In that principle, I explain the **physical addiction** of sugar and I also talk about the **psychological addiction**, including social pressure, bad habits, hormones, and obsessions.

In the same way you can re-educate your tastes and habits to like less fatty foods, you can change your desire for sugary foods. When people from other countries come to the United States, they are surprised by how sweet things taste here. Cereals, cookies, and drinks are sometimes so sweet that even their children can't eat them. Once they've been in the US for a while, they become used to the extra sugar. They re-educate their taste buds in the wrong direction.

Finding products that are low in sugar without falling into the trap of eating artificially sweetened food is difficult. (We talked about artificial sweeteners in **Step 3: Drinks**.) If you want a quality product that is low in sugar but not artificially sweetened, most of the time you will need to learn to cook it yourself. A good option is to use natural and organic ingredients, which tend to have lower sugar content without using artificial sweeteners, but be aware that many usually still have too much sugar.

The maximum 50 grams of sugar recommended by the WHO (much less the 25 grams that would be the optimum) is easy to get. Just a flavored yogurt can contain 20 to 25 grams of sugar! If you add the sugar in your tea or coffee, plus a cookie or a piece of chocolate, you are already at the maximum 50 grams recommended. This doesn't even include all the high carb foods (bread, corn chips, potatoes, etc.) that you eat daily. Remember, those are carbs that are easily transformed into simple sugars, so their effect is almost the same as simple sugar.

Remember: the best time to eat sugary products is after a main meal (lunch or dinner), never before the meal, and never alone as a snack, to avoid the high-glucose peak and the huge insulin response.

While everybody or almost everybody loves sugary products, **you need to learn to minimize them as much as possible, and always try to eat them with high fiber, whole grains and protein products to reduce the absorption.**

Importance of Fruit

Fruits contain large amounts of fructose. However, fructose is packed with fruit fiber and hence, this fiber buffers its absorption. This is why I recommended avoiding fruit juices where the fiber from the fruit has been eliminated—even the homemade ones!

Fructose is unable to generate a response to secrete leptin, and this is the reason I recommend eating fruit at the end of a meal. (See Principle 9 for more about leptin.) Once you have finished a meal, even though fructose does not activate leptin secretion, the other foods consumed during the meal will issue a response to secrete leptin and make you stop feeling hungry and start burning calories. If you have fruit as a snack, make sure you eat it with some source of protein (like cheese or ham).

Plus, fruit has many other nutritional benefits: it is packed with vitamins, minerals, and antioxidants, which are substances that may protect your cells from free radicals (free radicals are a consequence of exposure to chemicals, smoke, radiation, or pollution). The advantages of consuming fruit overcome the negatives of the sugar (fructose) it contains. It is better to limit the amount of sugar you add to your coffee, tea, yogurt, and other foods and cut out as many other hidden sources of fructose as you can than it is to eliminate fruit. Just don't overdo it; two servings of fruit per day are enough.

The Danger of High-Fructose Corn Syrup

In his book *The End of Overeating*, Dr. David A. Kessler writes that high-fructose corn syrup (HFCS) is a processed sweetener manufactured from the glucose in corn into fructose. Many foods in the United States contain HFCS because it is a cheap way to add sweetness to food. It has become common in many processed food including breads, meats, soups, and sauces to improve palatability.[24]

HFCS has replaced sucrose (or table sugar) for three main reasons: it is available and cheap compared to sucrose due to government subsidies of US corn[25], governmental production quotas of domestic sugar, and an import tax on foreign sugar[26].

Now you understand why high-fructose corn syrup is a cheap way to add sweetness to any processed food. The food industry found HFCS to be a gold mine, as it was a cost-effective way to increase our addiction not only to sweet food but also to the sugar-fat-salt combination in food. Adding HFCS allowed food manufacturers to improve the palatability of foods and therefore our addiction to those foods.

The main problem with HFCS is that because it is everywhere, you are eating a great deal of it without even realizing it. Get ten products from your kitchen cabinets or fridge and read the labels. Almost everything you eat on a daily basis contains HFCS.

The second problem with HFCS is that it seems to interfere with the mechanisms that make you feel full, and so you tend to eat more than necessary. There is a lot of controversy among researchers about what those mechanisms are, and the process is quite complicated, but the following explanation could be part of the reason:

› Fructose can only be processed in the liver[27] and does not stimulate insulin secretion from the pancreas,

› Insulin regulates the **leptin** response to meals, and

› **Leptin is the hormone that stops your sensation of hunger and activates calorie burning.**

Therefore, some researchers believe that a diet high in fructose inhibits leptin secretion, and as a result, you will eat more than necessary and will not burn many calories. In the long term, a diet high in HFCS may make you enter a cycle of weight and fat gain. It is not clear if a diet high in other types of sugars would lead to exactly the same effect, so my recommendation is to try to cut consumption of all sugars, and especially HFCS.

Some researchers even defend that high consumption of HFCS not only makes you fatter in general, but it makes you specifically accumulate more abdominal fat[28]. It seems the structure of HFCS versus the structure of sucrose (table sugar) could make the difference, because HFCS is more easily converted to fat than other sugars, leading to an easier body weight and fat gain, especially abdominal fat. But as I said, there is still a lot of controversy, and nothing has been scientifically proven yet.

Finally, you should know that HFCS is mostly manufactured from genetically modified corn, so eating HFCS is an easy way to introduce genetically modified organisms (GMOs) into your body. The full effects of genetically modified foods are not yet clear, but I would rather stay away from them since they are relatively new and negative effects have not been determined by scientists and researchers.

The Downside of Agave, Stevia, and Artificial Sweeteners

What I am most concerned in the 32 Mondays Weight Management Program is how artificial sweeteners interfere with sugar metabolism and increase sugar cravings and your appetite. You are probably wondering about agave and stevia, which are natural but concentrated sweeteners. Although no harmful effects have been detected yet, and the fact that they are natural makes me feel more comfortable, they are powerful and concentrated sweeteners. However, since they confuse your metabolism because they have few calories while your body is sensing a high calorie intake and altering your sugar taste, I recommend you avoid them as much as possible, just as with artificial sweeteners.

You have already learned about artificial sweeteners in **Step 3: Drinks**. They have been demonstrated to be harmful for your health. They can cause arthritis, gastrointestinal problems, and different types of cancer. Most importantly, they mess with your metabolism equilibrium, and you've already learned how important this is.

I would stay away from any artificial sweetener, even the newest ones. Scientific articles are continuously published about the negative effects of sweeteners. These sweeteners are like preservatives and colorants; they are not meant to be in our bodies. If you crave sweet flavors, learn how to control those cravings by feeding your body appropriately rather than feeding it with unhealthy artificial sweeteners, which just make you crave more sweets and more calories!

Cut Your Passion for Sugars

Cutting down on the sugar you eat can be quite challenging; here are some practical solutions for re-educating your taste buds and getting used to less sugar:

› Read labels and identify all sugar, especially the high-fructose corn syrup hidden in many products.

› Cut all direct sugar. Do you love coffee with loads of sugar? Use less each week until you get used to drinking it without sugar. This may take some time, but just the purity of coffee's flavor makes it worthwhile.

› Are you a candy lover who enjoys all the gummies, candy canes, and other sugary beauties on sale? Forget about them! They are 100 percent sugar with nothing added to help reduce its direct absorption (like fiber, fat, or protein), and they make your insulin mechanisms go haywire. Throw the rest to the garbage!

› Love cereals in the morning? Forget about the ones you see in commercials. Go for the organic ones—whole grain, high protein, high fiber if possible—with nothing added. Add just some fruit—blueberries, strawberries, blackberries, bananas—and some low-fat milk or yogurt and some granola if you need it a little bit sweeter.

› Substitute the candy bars you used to have for your after-meal treats with pure chocolate (the higher the percentage of cacao, the better).

› Cook or bake your own sweets using 50 percent of the suggested amount of sugar.

› Eat all sweets after your main meals. Mixing sweets with other nutrients, such as fiber, will stop the direct absorption of sugar.

› Choose an ice cream brand with a lower content of sugar.

› Go for unsweetened yogurts, milk, and other dairy.

› Avoid all drinks with added sugar.

› Avoid fruit juices or drink them with the fruit pulp.

› Avoid artificial sweeteners.

› Limit yourself to two servings of fruit per day, and eat it after a meal or as a snack with some protein or fat.

SUGGESTED TIME FRAME

You have four weeks, which is more than enough time to learn how bad direct sugar is and how to avoid it as much as possible. I know sugar has been your addiction for a long time, but it is time to break it. Physical addiction to nicotine, one of the most powerful addictions, lasts three to four days. Sugar is a much milder addiction than nicotine. Just stay away from it for a few days and use the four weeks to work on your mind and your psychological addiction. Read labels to avoid sugars and HFCS. Stop buying candies and candy bars, and throw away any you have—including that secret stash. Buy ingredients to cook your own treats or buy organic mixes to make treats with (usually) less sugar. Learn how to drink your coffee or tea without sugar. I promise you can do it!

TAKE 5

› **Learn**: Understand how sugars interact with your metabolism.

› **Goal**: Minimize the consumption of sugars.

› **Plan**: Substitute high sugary food with low- or no-sugar substitutes.

› **Monitor**: Maintain your food journal.

› **Reward**: Enjoy a nice variety of fresh fruit and sweet mix of berries every week.

KEY POINTS

› You eat too much sugar.

› Sugar is addictive.

› You can re-educate your taste for sugar.

› High-fructose corn syrup (HFCS) and other sugars are hidden in most processed foods.

› Artificial sweeteners are not healthy and should be avoided.

› Fruit is okay in moderation and eaten with other food rich in protein.

› Some sugar and treats are okay, but at the end of a meal.

STEP 8
CARBOHYDRATES

SUGGESTED TIME FRAME: 4 WEEKS

In **Step 7: Sugars**, you learned about basic sugars. Carbohydrates are sugars but with more complex structures. If you were using Lego blocks to build a carbohydrate, each block would be a basic sugar. When the blocks of sugar are linked to more and more basic sugars to form a long chain, you then have a carbohydrate.

Another analogy can be made with paper clips. A basic sugar is like a paper clip you use to keep paper together. When you build a long chain of clips, that's a carbohydrate. The longer the chain, the longer it will take to undo the chain, and you might even leave the clips bound together. When you stick papers in between the clips, the chain becomes more difficult to undo. In our analogy, those papers are the fiber in a complex carbohydrate.

To absorb food, your body needs to break it down until it becomes basic forms—like Lego pieces or paper clips, or basic sugars. The longer the carbohydrate chains, the longer it will take to break the chain and the longer food will remain in your body, sending the signal that you still have food available and therefore you don't need more—meaning you don't feel hungry. Not only that, but to break those chains, you need to expend energy. The longer and more complex the chain, the higher the energy expenditure needed.

When you eat simple sugars (any sugary product like candies or cookies), your body doesn't need to do any work to absorb it, so the process happens quickly and you feel empty and hungry again in a short period of time. When you eat longer-chain carbohydrates like rice, wheat, bread, and pasta, your body takes longer to process them so you feel full for a longer period, plus your body expends energy in the processing of those calories.

When you eat carbohydrates that are made from whole grains, the process works still more in your favor. Whole grains have fiber, which is difficult to break; most of it will never be broken nor absorbed. Slowing the absorption process means a longer time of not feeling hungry. Fiber makes the absorption of basic sugars more difficult and adds zero additional calories to your meal because fiber does not have calories. Plus, the process requires plenty of calories. All benefits! This is what happens when you eat whole-wheat or whole-grain bread, pasta, cookies, and muffins, and brown rice instead of white. Fiber is also the reason it is better to eat whole fruits instead juices. Whole fruits have all the fiber in them to slow the absorption of the sugars in the fruit, plus fiber makes you feel full for a longer time. Juices have the fiber from the fruit removed, so they provide direct sugars that are quickly absorbed.

If you have a choice, go for whole-grain bread instead of whole-wheat bread because it has more soluble fiber and therefore a lower glycemic index (GI) and glycemic load (GL). This is an important concept for weight management. If you are interested in learning a bit more about it you can get my free e-book at my website, *www.32mondays.com*.

Other important examples of better choices related to GI and GL are to have sweet potatoes instead of white potatoes, barley instead of rice, and couscous or quinoa instead of pasta. And go for nuts and beans—they've had bad press because they are high in calories, but the GI and GL are low, and they are perfect foods if you respect the portion sizes. Brown rice, although it has better numbers than white rice, still has higher than desirable GI and GL values, so try to eat it only from time to time and always respect the serving size of one cup.

Not only are whole grains good for your weight management, but they are packed with vitamins and minerals that are extremely important for your health. In addition, although the link between high-fiber diets and cancer risk is inconclusive, "Research *is* clear that eating a high-fiber diet can help you stay at a healthy weight, which in turn, lowers your risk for many kinds of cancer," according to WebMD.com.[29] Again, all benefits!

Getting used to whole grains is important and easy for weight management. The only thing you need to change is to choose whole grains whenever possible. The taste *is* different, but believe me, once you get used to the full taste of whole grains, you will never want to go back to the plain and tasteless ones.

How to Move to Whole Wheat and Whole Grains

To move from the white enemies to the whole-grain allies, you need to organize your approach. I suggest you start by changing your treats. You can even add a few more treats to your diet to help you appreciate the whole-grain varieties. It is quite difficult to find healthy, whole-grain treats like muffins and cookies, and you need to be careful they don't have bad fats added. You might find it easier to bake them at home, although remember to read the ingredient labels. I would recommend cooking a batch of delicious oat muffins or cookies, and start switching to whole grains with those. You can freeze what you don't immediately need.

Then move to whole-grain breads—so tasty, believe me! After that, move to brown rice, which generally takes longer to cook (forty-five to fifty-five minutes). You'll need to get organized in advance when you want to have brown rice. Consider cooking enough for the whole week to avoid waiting every time you want to eat rice. You can find precooked or quick-cooking cereals like farro, bulgur, and barley, and even almost-instant brown rice that cooks in ten minutes! There is even precooked, frozen brown rice that is ready after three minutes in the microwave.

Don't forget about quinoa and couscous, which are perfect companions for any stir-fry and are super easy, fast to cook, and have only a medium glycemic index and glycemic load.

The final change should be pasta. We are so used to white pasta that this might be the most difficult change for you, especially because of the different whole-wheat pasta texture. There are brands now for whole-wheat tortellini, which could be a good starting point. Then move to whole-wheat pasta and cook it with meat and tomato sauce to try to cover a bit of the whole-grain taste. Move to plain whole-wheat pasta once you have totally integrated all the whole-grain products. It can take you some time to get used to the whole-wheat pasta texture and flavor. You can cheat from time to time with white fiber pasta, which claims to have three times the fiber of regular white pasta.

If this step is difficult for you, just think how much better off you are now that you can eat whole-grain carbohydrates compared to all the diets you have followed that forbade almost all carbohydrates. If you haven't been on a diet that cut carbohydrates, just think how your body is benefiting from a change to whole-grain carbs. Not only are you moving toward keeping your weight under control, but you are getting all the benefits from eating extra fiber and all the vitamins and minerals from whole grains.

By the way, make sure the products are 100 percent whole-wheat or grain. Check the label to be sure they have at least 3 grams of fiber per serving. Don't be fooled by misleading package marketing—read the label and check that whole-grain wheat or grain is the first ingredient.

Remember: carbohydrates are where we tend to overestimate the portion size. We often serve and eat double the portion size, which is only one cup, about the size of your fist.

SUGGESTED TIME FRAME

I allowed four weeks for this step because moving from conventional carbs to whole grain can be a real challenge for some people. The timing will go more or less like this:

> › **First week**: Choose whole-grain or whole-wheat treats: muffins, cookies, or bagels. Remember to check for low sugar and low fat!

> › **Second week**: Move to whole-grain, whole-wheat breads. Choose whole wheat as a first ingredient, with a minimum 3 grams of fiber per serving, plus low sugar, low fat!

› **Third week**: Replace rice with couscous, quinoa, bulgur, farro, barley, and brown rice occasionally.

› **Fourth week**: Move to whole-wheat pasta.

TAKE 5

› **Learn**: Understand that carbohydrates are a complex form of sugars, and that whole-wheat and whole-grain forms are much better for your metabolism.

› **Goal**: Minimize your consumption of refined carbohydrates and move to whole wheat and whole grains.

› **Plan**: Substitute "white" carbohydrates for "brown" ones.

› **Monitor**: Maintain the food journal.

› **Reward**: Keep a nice variety of whole-wheat pancakes and muffin mixes to bake at home.

KEY POINTS

› Whole-wheat and/or whole-grain bread, pasta, and cereals are complex carbohydrates that stay longer in your system and give you a feeling of satiation for a longer period.

› Fiber is free of calories and reduces the absorption of fat and simple sugars.

› Your body spends energy digesting fiber.

› Whole wheat/whole grains are good for insulin equilibrium and colon health.

› Your treats will have less impact on your weight if they are whole wheat or whole grain.

› Organize the switch into whole-grain products one week/one group at a time.

› Rice is not a good option because of its high GI and GL. Have it in moderation, and always choose brown instead of white.

› As always, read labels carefully. "Contains whole grains" is not the same as 100 percent whole wheat or whole grain. For maximum benefit, whole grain should be the first ingredient listed.

› Look for at least 2 to 3 grams of fiber per serving.

› Don't get fooled by misleading food labels stating "healthy" food. Read the actual composition on the label.

STEP 9
SALT

Here we are again. Remember the highly palatable food in the fat-sugar-salt combination? The food manufacturing industry is reaping the benefits again, this time by manipulating sodium, especially in snacks and ready-to-eat convenience foods.

Salty food is not only tastier but also more addictive. You get hooked on salty food, and therefore you have stronger cravings and you eat more. You especially eat more of the nasty combo foods: high salt, high fat, and high sugar. Salty foods are usually high in fats, too, especially hydrogenated fats.

Consumption of excess salt makes you retain liquids. The reason is a biological process called osmosis. When too much salt enters your body, your kidneys have to let more water into the bloodstream to neutralize the salt excess and make it in equilibrium with the rest of your body. When more water is in your blood it makes your blood pressure rise (more volume, more pressure).

High blood pressure increases the risk of heart disease and stroke. Also your kidneys, arteries, heart, and brain suffer negative effects when you have a diet high in salt[30]. While the government recommends only one teaspoon a day (2,300 milligrams), 70 percent of the population in the United States is at risk of developing health problems associated to a high consumption of salt. Ninety percent of the adult population will develop high blood pressure at some point in their lives[31].

Directly related to our weight management objective here, a high-salt diet is associated with more and bigger fat cells in the body.

There aren't many options to fight high consumption of salt other than to cut back. The same principles and recommendations I've made about sugar can be applied to salt addiction. Again, please go back to **Principle 7: Physical and Psychological Food Addictions in Part I of the book where I discuss addiction**.

Some Recommendations to Help You Consume Less Salt

The first thing to do is to avoid all salty snacks (chips, crackers, corn chips, salty nuts) and packaged, cooked meals, which are usually saturated with salt. Avoid them completely if you can, or look for the reduced-salt products.

You need to re-educate your taste buds step-by-step and get used to eating less salt. Once you have learned to avoid salty foods, you should get used to adding less salt to your own food. Never, ever add salt before tasting a meal, and start substituting the many spices you have available so you won't miss the salt you're used to. Celery flakes, garlic and onion powder, pepper, and many herbs and spices are good allies to help you reduce the amount of salt you are consuming. Don't be tricked by flavored salts (garlic, onion, celery, and others) which often contain more sodium than table salt! And be careful with herb and seasoning mixes because many of them contain too much salt.

By now, you should be cooking or preparing most of your foods with healthy ingredients. By avoiding prepared meals, you're already avoiding a high amount of salt.

SUGGESTED TIME FRAME

Unfortunately, many people are not aware of the negatives of a diet high in salt or of the short- and long-term consequences associated with high blood pressure. Even if they have a notion of the health risks, they don't do anything until they receive a diagnosis of high blood pressure, are put on medication to lower their blood pressure, and are told to restrict their salt intake.

One of the major problems with salt as I explained before is that it is added to many of the manufactured foods to increase palatability, make you addicted to that food, and to use as a preservative. As a consequence, just by eating processed foods the majority of Americans are consuming too much salt.

By following the 32 Mondays Weight Management Program, you are eliminating most processed foods and the amount of salt in your diet, and therefore reducing the risks of high blood pressure and its associated health problems.

Even with the salt we consume with a diet free of highly processed foods, we are consuming enough salt to supply our needs. With just some veggies, cheese, and bread we have enough sodium. By adding a pinch of salt to our meals, we are more than covered!

On the other hand, if you eat a diet totally free of processed foods and you eat with no added salt, you can end up having a deficit and, as a consequence, low blood pressure, which can give you a problem like dizziness. So be careful if you plan to follow a low-sodium diet.

Just accept how bad high salt consumption is for you. Cut salty foods right now, and reduce how much salt you add to your meals. Avoid salty snacks, add and cook with less salt, and use more herbs and spices instead. Come on, just do it! Only one week here!

TAKE 5

› **Learn**: Understand why salt is bad for you and where is hidden in most foods.

› **Goal**: Minimize the consumption of salt.

› **Plan**: Reduce salt intake by checking labels for hidden salt in most food as well as reducing the amount of salt used in cooking and eating.

> **Monitor**: Check the food journal.

> **Reward**: Treat yourself to a manual salt grinder to always remind you not to add too much salt to your food.

KEY POINTS

> Salt, especially salty food, is addictive.

> Salt is part of the fat-sugar-salt trio the food manufacturing industry uses to manipulate buying decisions.

> A diet high in salt makes you retain water and generate more fat cells, and increases the risk of certain serious diseases.

> Commercial snacks and processed meals are packed with extra salt.

> When cooking, use spices to reduce the amount of salt you add to the meal.

STEP 10
ALCOHOL

A lot has been written about alcoholic drinks, but there is not a total and general agreement on the benefits or risks. For some doctors and dieticians, it is something to avoid completely, while for others, a drink could be beneficial to your body. What all experts agree with is that an excess amount of alcohol is bad for your body and is packed with calories.

Alcohol is considered a form of sugar in terms of how it is processed by your body. Calories derived from alcohol are technically empty calories. This means from a strictly nutritional point of view, alcohol does not give your body anything beneficial that can be used by your body. **Alcohol in your body is metabolized as a sugar and transformed easily into fat, especially into visceral or abdominal fat**.

Benefits of Alcohol

The truth is that recent studies and investigations suggest there are certain components of alcohol that can be beneficial to your body[32]. Those components protect your heart and arteries and work in your favor by protecting you from certain heart diseases, helping to raise good cholesterol (HDL). Those components also help with fat management and even with sugar management in the blood by assisting insulin. All these benefits are there *as long as you stay with one drink per day for women and two for men.*

Some time ago it was believed that only red wine could provide us with the benefits from the positive antioxidant effects of tannins and resveratrol [33]. As I said before, new studies have demonstrated that it is the alcohol per se that gives those benefits, not any other ingredient. Of course, this idea could change at any moment when more results from further investigation are obtained, but at present, this is what you should consider as true.

For some people, alcohol has some psychological benefit. Our optimal well-being is important to be able to maintain a healthy lifestyle, and your well-being is important for you to be able to follow the steps in this Program.

Therefore, alcohol is allowed under these specific conditions:

› *Only one drink per day for women and two for men.* This is the quantity currently suggested by the scientific community to maintain the benefits without deriving undesirable health effects[34].

› *Drink only after eating.* When you drink on an empty stomach, the effect of the alcohol is two or more times stronger than when you drink after having some food in your stomach. This is because food acts as an absorbent, stopping the effect of alcohol in your body. When you drink on an empty stomach, your willpower is easily overpowered, which can lead you to forget about your eating "norms" learned in this program. Wait until you have eaten something; the best moment to have a drink is when you are in the middle of a meal. Remember, the alcohol affects your body the same as sugar, therefore the insulin reaction when having it by itself is the same as if you'd had a sugary snack.

› *What to drink.* Of course I am not going to tell you what to drink! But I will give some details of the calorie contents of certain drinks, and even a tip about how many calories you are saving if you move to lighter drinks. Remember, if you mix your drink with any soft and sugary drink, you need to consider those extra calories.

And by the way, remember to keep note of your drinks in your food diary! Drinks count!

Beverage	Calories
beer (12 oz)	150
light beer (12 oz)	100
wine, red or white (5 oz) 1 glass	100
gin, rum, vodka, whiskey (one shot)	100
martini, bloody mary	120
gin & tonic, screwdriver	200
mai tai, margarita, sweet wine	350
mudslide	800

So think twice when you choose your drink!

Some Tips to Help You Go Easy on Alcoholic Drinks

› Start by being aware of what are you drinking. Count the number of drinks and write them in your journal. Look back at the journal and decide where you have to cut.

› Leave drinks for dinner. Consider them treats, and only have them if you have behaved during the day.

› Never drink on an empty stomach and wait to start your drink until you have started eating your main meal.

› Decide what you are drinking and stay there. Switching drinks makes you drink more. The more variety, the more you eat and drink.

› Try to avoid sugary, mixed alcoholic drinks. Not only does the alcohol add calories, but so does the mixer.

SUGGESTED TIME FRAME

You have one week to change your approach to alcohol. If you are used to having crazy alcoholic weekends, you need to reconsider them and instead view alcohol as a tasting pleasure, not an out-of-control action. Cut the amount to one drink per day, maximum two for men. Your approach to alcohol has to be similar to your approach to salt and sugar: you have to believe it is bad, and just stop doing it!

TAKE 5

> **Learn**: Understand why only a small amount of alcohol is good for you.

> **Goal**: Drink a maximum of one drink a day for women and two for men.

> **Plan**: Decide what and when you are going to have your drink(s).

> **Monitor**: Include all alcoholic beverages in your food journal.

> **Reward**: Treat yourself to a nice wine glass or beer mug.

KEY POINTS

> Alcohol is empty calories.

> Metabolically, alcohol is a sugar.

> Too much alcohol will be transformed into visceral or abdominal fat.

> Research suggests certain health benefits from one drink of alcohol per day for women, two for men.

> Drink after you have started your meal.

> Not all drinks are created equal; choose lower-calorie alcoholic beverages whenever possible.

> Drinks count: add them to your food diary.

STEP 11
VIGOROUS EXERCISE

SUGGESTED TIME FRAME: 4 WEEKS

In Step 2, you started a program of moderate exercise. The objective was to make you get off your couch, start a more active lifestyle, and help you start losing weight. In this step, you are getting serious about exercise, and you will embark on a program you should be able to maintain for life.

Even if you already practice vigorous exercise, there are still many things you can learn in this chapter to obtain the most benefit from an intense exercise program, especially from the weight loss point of view. Please remember: if you are not currently involved in a physical activity program, check with your physician before enrolling in one.

Benefits of Vigorous Exercise

I can't describe all the benefits you can derive from day one from engaging in a program of vigorous exercise, but I'll mention some of the most important.

Psychologically, you will feel empowered. You will feel like you can be and do better. When you exercise vigorously, you secrete *endorphins*, a hormone that helps you enormously to feel better. It is like a happy hormone, and it is addictive, a good addiction. This feeling will help you follow the right pathway on your weight management journey.

Physically, you will feel stronger day by day, even when you feel tired from exercising. You will feel more and more energetic. Your body shape will improve, and you will spend more calories exercising and feeding those extra muscles, which will help in your weight management. Several hormones related to your weight management system are released while performing high-intensity exercise, including growth hormone. Not only that, but the effect of the hormones secreted during the intense exercise lasts for an hour after an aerobic exercise like running and up to forty-eight hours after a strengthening session like weight lifting. Your body's metabolic rate rises during exercise and for hours afterward.

Now, if you want to know more specific benefits of exercising, here is a list:

> promotes weight loss and decreases appetite

> controls insulin peaks and helps prevent type 2 diabetes

> decreases the risk of heart disease and stroke and the development of hypertension

> lowers the risk of osteoporosis and breast and colon cancer

> helps prevent arthritis and maintain healthy joints

> increases the levels of:

  ○ glutathione, the major antioxidant in cells, which slows down the overall aging process

  ○ dopamine, related to motivation, drive, and stimulation

  ○ serotonin, which provides feelings of peace and happiness

  ○ endorphins, which provides pleasure feelings and eliminates pain

> helps you attain restful sleep

> › improves digestion

> › helps prevent colds and flu

Both the physical and the psychological effects will most likely end up as sort of a need for you, and you will feel the need to exercise for your well-being.

Exercise for Weight Loss

I have never considered exercise the only way to lose weight. Although exercise has a lot to do with weight management (because it promotes weight loss and decreases appetite), it is difficult to count only on exercise to lose weight. Believe me, you shouldn't enroll in one of those mega-vigorous programs of intense exercise that not many of us, not even the already fit, would be able to maintain. It is true that when you exercise you burn more calories than when you do not, but when you exercise in excess, you end up overtired and unable to make the right decisions on weight management, and too hungry to apply common sense when choosing the right foods. Therefore, be careful about over-exercising.

The truth is, it is difficult to lose weight by only exercising, and it is difficult to exercise when you are overweight. That is why vigorous exercise begins during one of the last weeks of the 32 Mondays Weight Management Program. By now, you should have lost enough weight to be able to exercise more freely, without too many extra pounds or kilograms hindering your movements. When you engage in a vigorous exercise program, you will benefit from the psychological effects, which will help you stay on the right path. You will start to define your body shape, which will enhance your well-being, and you will burn more calories as you build more muscle. A muscular body is not only nicer than a fat body, but it also burns many more calories, even when resting. Your basal metabolism (the energy you consume only to maintain the basics of your body at rest) increases, and your active metabolism increases still more. All this extra burning effect will help you lose the extra weight you want to lose and then maintain your desired weight.

Incorporate Exercise into Your Life

Vigorous exercise is hard to do and hard to maintain. No matter how fit you already are and how good the benefits are, it is always easier to sit down in front of the TV or the computer, or have a cup of coffee with a friend, than it is to exercise. This is the reason you *really* need to incorporate it into your routine. Consider exercise as important as brushing your teeth, bringing the kids to school, or going to work. You should decide the best time of the day and the best days of the week to exercise. Some trainers recommend a specific time of the day (usually evenings) to increase the beneficial effects and the burning results. To me, the most important thing is to find a time that works best for you and maintain it.

I recommend three days of vigorous exercise per week, two days during the week and one over the weekend. The idea is to consider those two week-days as days you can't skip, and then have one activity over the weekend to complete the three days. I would recommend finding a fun activity over the weekend to really enjoy and appreciate your exercise. I think that's a realistic amount of exercise for the super-busy person you are.

Aging

You may think, "I am getting older, I am not fit for a vigorous exercise any-more, leave it for the young ones." Bad news: the older you get, the more you need to follow a vigorous exercise routine. Adults lose between a half pound (226 grams) and one pound (450 grams) of muscle tissue every year after the age of twenty-five. That means every ten years you burn between 100 and 400 fewer calories each day. Our bodies naturally progress toward more fat and less muscle, which means a decrease in our metabolism rate or calorie burn. You need to work harder to fight the natural tendency to lose muscle and gain fat[35]. Hey, ladies, this is especially true for you because women have less total muscle than men[36]. So, if you never thought about it before, now is the time to get serious about exercising.

Here's the good news: for each pound (450 Grams) of muscle mass you either gain or keep from losing, you will burn approximately 50 to 100 calories a day, which you can use toward achieving your weight objective or to indulge yourself with a treat if you are already at your desired weight.

Types of Vigorous Exercise

In my mind, the best exercise you can ever practice is the one you like and feel motivated enough to do. The truth is, as I mentioned before, it is hard to practice vigorous exercise. If you want to maintain its practice, you need to find one you like that is convenient. If you choose skiing, which is a great exercise, it can be only practiced in winter and most likely over the weekend, so you'll need to include other exercises for the rest of the time.

For optimum results, choose two types of vigorous exercise, one aerobic and one strengthening activity.

Aerobic exercise, also called cardio, is exercise with an intensity low enough for the body to still maintain the normal supply of oxygen to the cells. Simply by breathing deeply and faster and making your heart work harder, you are able to maintain your activity without hurting your body.

An aerobic exercise maintained at a moderate pace for twenty minutes is the fat-burning exercise par excellence.

Running at a pace that allows you to breathe normally, meaning you are able to talk but not sing, is the aerobic exercise I always recommend. It is excellent for burning calories, helps develop a long and lean musculature, and greatly improves your heart functioning, among other benefits. The best thing about running is you can practice it wherever you are, and you only need your running shoes. You don't need to run a marathon, although participating in races is encouraging and motivating. If you find running difficult, start little by little, adding some more distance every day. The idea is to build up to running for twenty to thirty minutes, two to three times a week, and increase your speed over time. If you still have to lose a lot of weight to feel comfortable, you have joint or balance problems, or feel uncomfortable running given your current health, just find another vigorous exercise that fits you better.

Swimming is another excellent exercise—if you have access to a pool, of course. If you like the idea of swimming, go for it.

Biking requires either a bike or a gym with static bikes. Be careful if you are concerned about developing your lower extremities too much. Contrary to what you would think, if you practice long vigorous cycling sessions too many days a week, you can develop your lower extremities more than desired.

Other aerobic exercises include aerobic dancing, water aerobics, cardio yoga, kickboxing, or using stair stepping and elliptical machines, among others. You'll need a gym or similar if you decide to engage in one of those programs, but exercising in a group is easier for some people.

Sports like basketball, soccer, tennis, volleyball, racquetball, and similar activities are other aerobic exercises. You may also enjoy outdoor exercises such as skiing (cross country or alpine), kayaking, hiking, climbing, and skating. In general, any exercise you practice outdoors will double the benefits as you also get fresh air and sunlight, which helps improve your well-being, and you spend more energy regulating your body temperature when it's cold or hot outside.

Anaerobic exercise is any short-lasting, high-intensity activity, like yoga or Pilates, that relies on energy stored in the muscles and is not dependent on oxygen. Strength or weight training are the anaerobic exercises par excellence.

My recommendation is to wait to start a strength-training program until after you have lost enough weight to feel comfortable exercising, changed some eating behaviors, and started a moderate exercise routine so you feel more flexible and strong enough to start a strength-training program. If you start with a vigorous program of weight lifting before losing some weight, you will find yourself developing muscles before losing the fat, adding more and more volume to your body. That said, if you have followed my time schedule, by now you should have lost some weight, and you are probably ready for your strength-training session.

Strength Training

Strength training includes weight training with machines or free weights, resistance-band activities, and balance-ball activities. It is excellent for weight loss because it helps you maintain and develop muscle mass, which helps increase your metabolism and decrease body fat. Strength training also improves the cell's sensitivity to insulin, so the insulin metabolism will be better regulated. It is important to develop muscles because they burn much more energy than simple fat. Remember that one pound (450 grams) of muscle burns between 50 and 100 calories. Also, when you are losing weight, 25 percent of the weight loss is in the form of muscle, and therefore you need to recover it.

Muscles are your own internal energy-burning machine that work constantly, even when you are not active. When those muscles are under activity, they burn more calories. Also, while strength training, the muscles involved are micro-injured, which means your body expends more energy in the healing process. An additional benefit of strength training is it helps shape your body. Don't worry about developing bulky muscles— you would need several hours of strenuous weight lifting every day to build them.

To eliminate the risk of injury, you need to maintain good posture and form during the exercises and learn the correct lifting techniques, motion, breaths, and speed of movement. If you don't know them, hire a personal trainer or enroll in a group class. Strength training videos from the Mayo Clinic can help you learn the right way to perform exercises: http://www.mayoclinic. org/healthy-lifestyle/fitness/in-depth/strength-training/art-20046031.

Pilates

No matter how much you exercise per week and how fit you are, Pilates is an essential exercise. Pilates gives you strength in the core of your body—the central area around the tummy and lower back. When the core of the body becomes strong, you are much better able to cope with other types of exercise. Plus, your posture improves dramatically, resulting in a better figure and more well-being—and with less back pain. Sometimes, a whole hour of class becomes tedious, sometimes even boring. Fifteen-minute sessions with the most effective exercises, two to three times a week is enough to maintain your good shape. Plus, you can practice Pilates anywhere. You only need a gym mat or a couple of folded towels on the floor. If you have never practiced Pilates before, you can enroll in private or group lessons. Once you have learned the basic movements, you can practice them on your own. If you have experience practicing floor exercises, there are also good books with photos, diagrams, and explanations that can guide you through the learning curve.

The 32 Mondays Vigorous Exercise Program

Your intensive exercise program starts with strength exercises to consume all the glycogen stored in your liver and muscles after your last meal and then goes to the aerobic exercise to burn stored fat once no more glycogen is available.

Although some experts recommend aerobic exercise first followed by strength training so you won't be too tired for the aerobic activity, if your goal is maximum weight loss, you need to consume the glycogen first so you will burn the stored fat later.

Appendix C contains a list of calories burned in thirty minutes of completing various exercises. Keep in mind the idea of a vigorous exercise is not only to burn calories to lose weight, but to increase your metabolism, build muscles, and to release more weight management-friendly hormones to help you burn calories more efficiently.

Preparing to Exercise: Meals and the Energy Bar Trap

Make sure you have had a good meal no more than two or three hours prior to your exercise routine. If that's not possible, have a healthy snack thirty minutes to an hour before you begin so you'll have energy for the workout. It is not a good idea to work out when you are hungry, since you will burn muscle to get energy for your workout. Muscle is what you are trying to build.

Please, plan your meals according to your exercise routines and leave the energy snacks and drinks to the athletes. Energy bars contain at least 12 grams of sugar. Most conventional bars have 20 to 30 grams each. When you drink an energy drink or eat an energy bar while exercising, you are adding an important amount of sugar to your system. Not only are you adding calories, but you are having a sugar snack, stimulating an insulin peak with its consequences, and by not depleting your sugar resources, you'll enter the fat burning mode much later. And to put things in perspective, one of those bars or a sugary drink equates to one hour of walking or thirty minutes of intense running or cycling.

Finally, and very important: wait thirty minutes to eat after a workout to take advantage of your body's fat-burning ability. Your body is using stored fat as fuel because all the immediate glucose and glycogen have already been consumed. If you eat immediately after your workout, you provide easy fuel so the body will stop burning fat for energy. If you wait for thirty minutes, you will keep burning fat until your body realizes it needs glucose to keep going, and then the brain will release ghrelin to make you feel hungry and make you eat.

Intensity of Exercise

Every activity you choose can be performed at a different level of intensity. Your target rate zone varies depending on your age and your level of fitness. I will explain here how to calculate the recommended training for optimal fat burning and muscle building depending on your age. You can choose whether to work out at the minimum or maximum Training Pulse Rate (TPR) according to how you feel and how confident you are that you can achieve the upper level without overdoing it.

TRAINING PULSE RATE (TPR) FOR FAT BURNING

> › MHR is the maximum heart rate

> › TPR is the training pulse rate

For fat burning purposes with practicing aerobic exercise, a TPR in the 65 to 85 percent zone of your MHR is recommended; MHR is calculated by subtracting your age from 220.

MHR: 220 minus your age

Minimum TPR for Fat burning = MHR x 65%

Maximum TPR for Fat burning = MHR x 85%

So, if you are forty-two years old:

MHR: 220 – 42 = 178

Minimum TPR = 178 x 0.65 = 116 beats per minute

Maximum TPR = 178 X 0.85 = 142 beats per minute

The Training Pulse Rate is an easy formula to use and remember;

however, it is not totally accurate as it doesn't take into account your fitness status, which can be measured by your heartbeats per minute when resting. To take into account your present fitness status, use the Lagerstrom equation to calculate training pulse rate. This formula considers your fat-burning zone is between 60 percent and 70 percent of the maximum heart rate after considering your resting pulse (RP).

$$\text{MHR: 220 minus your age}$$

$$\text{Factor X} = \text{MHR minus RP}$$

$$\text{Lower TPR} = 0.6 \text{ Factor X} + \text{RP}$$

$$\text{Upper TPR} = 0.7 \text{ Factor X} + \text{RP}$$

If the same forty-two-year-old person mentioned above hasn't exercised in a long time and has a resting pulse of 72 beats per minute:

$$\text{MHR} = 220 - 42 = 178$$

$$\text{Factor X: } 178 - 72 = 106$$

$$\text{Lower TPR} = (0.6 \times 106) + 72 = 136$$

$$\text{Upper TPR} = (0.7 \times 106) + 72 = 146$$

If, on the contrary, the person is well-trained and exercises regularly, and her resting pulse is 55:

$$\text{MHR} = 220 - 42 = 178$$

$$\text{Factor X: } 178 - 55 = 123$$

$$\text{Lower TPR} = (0.6 \times 123) + 55 = 129$$

$$\text{Upper TPR} = (0.7 \times 123) + 55 = 141$$

You should work out in the upper or lower levels of the range depending on the type of exercise you are practicing. If you are running, skating, or cross-country skiing at a fast pace, you should work out in the upper limit. If you are cycling or practicing another exercise at a moderate pace, you should work in the middle area. Work out in the lower range if you are swimming or practicing aquatic gymnastics.

STAGES

These four stages of your vigorous exercise program focus on fat burning and weight loss. You should include all four stages for optimal results.

> **Stage 1: Warm-Up**
>
> Use five minutes to stretch and warm up your body. You don't need to do anything too specific, and you don't want to get tired from the warm-up. Climbing some stairs or a short walk can do it.

> **Stage 2: Strengthening**

- Practice twenty to thirty minutes of strengthening exercises (free weights, machines, or Pilates). Make sure to pay attention to how you perform each movement, and maintain the right posture. It is important to focus and visualize the muscles you are working out to get the best results.

- You should typically perform ten to twelve repetitions per set. If you are just starting your program, perform only one set and increase to two to three sets per activity once you become better conditioned over time. Go for more repetitions and sets after some time to keep improving.

- Minimize rests between repetitions to maximize the burning effect.

- Do two exercises with the same muscle group and then switch to another group, alternating upper and lower body muscle groups.

- Do not do the same exercises every day. Let the muscles have time to repair and rebuild; leave one or two days between workouts.

- Change the exercises from time to time to develop other muscles and add variety to your workout and avoid getting bored.

  In this phase, you will burn the available glycogen (stored sugar) in the muscle and liver so you enter into Stage 3 with no glycogen and are therefore able to burn stored fat during your moderate aerobic exercise.

› **Stage 3: Fat-Burning Aerobic Routine**

In order to burn fat as fuel, you should maintain an aerobic activity for at least twenty to thirty minutes.

If you are new to aerobic exercise, start by working out in a low heart rate range of the TPR you have calculated according to your age and current fitness status. Increase gradually to the upper level once you become more aerobically conditioned.

Remember that aerobic means *in the presence of oxygen*, which means you should be able to breathe air (oxygen) naturally; you should be able to talk but not sing. When you exercise to the point you are short of breath, you are no longer performing aerobically but anaerobically. Anaerobic exercise burns glycogen (stored sugar) rather than fat. As the glycogen has been previously consumed in Stage 2, if you work out anaerobically, you will start burning muscle protein as a fuel for your workout instead of fat.

Also, if you are overweight or obese and you work out at an intensity higher than your normal pace (talking but not singing), you may increase your cortisol levels (stress hormone), which facilitates the accumulation of body fat.

○ If you need or like to work out in the morning before breakfast, you can use the benefits of the night hormones to extend the fat-burning process occurring at night. If you choose to do so, it is extremely important you perform only Stage 3, and for about twenty minutes, to avoid using muscle protein to maintain your strength workout.

› **Stage 4: Cool Down**

Cool down by practicing a moderate aerobic exercise and stretching for five minutes. Take some time to relax and reconnect with yourself after the exercise.

High-Intensity Interval Training

A specific way of exercising that requires a separate mention, which you can incorporate or not according to your specific preferences, is high-intensity interval training (HIIT). It mixes high-intensity bursts of exercise with moderate-intensity recovery periods, usually for less than twenty minutes. Do not start HIIT until you have been practicing vigorous exercise for a few months and you are reasonably fit.

Various studies in recent years have proven that high-intensity interval training or cross training is an effective way to improve overall cardiovascular health and your ability to burn fat faster[37].

To perform your HIIT while practicing your aerobic routine, you should aim to reach almost your maximum capacity while exercising, not during the entire routine but in certain peaks for a duration of about ten seconds.

Exercise Maintenance

My last word is about *maintenance*. Starting a new program of vigorous exercise can be difficult. It is much easier to maintain something once than to leave it and have to start from zero again. To use a business analogy, it is always worth the effort to maintain an old client than to get a new one. Similarly, it is easier to maintain your present physical strength and routine than it is to start over again. If you need to take a few days off for any reason, just resume your exercise routine as soon as you can. In the meantime, when you can't keep your normal routine, try to find a substitute. Maybe you can walk or swim with your kids, double the use of your stairs at home, start using the stairs at work, or look for a vacation where you can plan some exercise. There are always ways to increase your basal activity.

Practical Ways to Start a Vigorous Exercise Program: Friends and Family

There are many types of vigorous exercises you can enjoy with someone else. Exercising together can make a relationship closer or give the whole family something in common to do.

Find a friend who already practices that activity or who is willing to start. If you can't find anybody to share your exercise, join a group. You'll be surprised how many groups for all fitness levels you can find in your community. Running, cycling, trekking, skating, climbing, skiing, and rowing are all examples of those activities.

Finding an activity you can practice with your family is a marvelous way to strengthen your relationship with them. We are used to taking our kids to team practices: ballet, ice skating, soccer, judo, and tennis lessons, but we usually don't practice anything together.

It is true that most activities require an investment, either to join a gym or to buy equipment like shoes, skis, climbing equipment, bikes, or skates. Sometimes you need to travel some distance with all the equipment, as with mountain biking or skiing. But the closeness you develop with your family when practicing a sport together is priceless. It is a precious time everyone enjoys together as you are all trying to get better at what you do, learning from each other, working as a team to prepare and organize the equipment or the trip, or face challenging difficulties like being cold, tired, thirsty, hungry, or scared. The happiness of your kids when they achieve something difficult and when you are directly there to help and support them is exceptional. Not only are you exercising, but you are also teaching your kids good and healthy habits like how to persist to improve, face challenges, and enjoy the achievements.

If you don't have kids, practicing a sport together brings a couple together, too. It is enjoyable to go out and buy new equipment, make mistakes, challenge one another, and even engage in some healthy competition. This is what memories are made of.

Tips for Success

› Plan. Plan your exercise days and times, and stay consistent every week if possible. Try to never plan another activity during those reserved days and times. If you travel a lot and you can't exercise during the week, try to find hotels with gyms. I once met a triathlete who travelled for business and took his static training bike with him everywhere.

› Just do it. Don't allow time for procrastination. If it is your planned exercise day and time, don't think, just go and do it!

› Think positively. Think about how well you feel after exercising, how much your overall performance improves, and even how your ability to think properly improves. Avoid the negative thinking like you are tired or have too many things to do.

› Set clear objectives per week, month, and year, and keep a journal of the objectives you accomplish. For example, for the strength-training routine, increase one repetition every day and one set every month until you reach your final objective. Increase the weight you use every month.

› Have fun! Find activities you enjoy, try to learn a new sport, and practice with family and friends as much as you can.

SUGGESTED TIME FRAME

You have four weeks to engage in a vigorous exercise program. During the first week, you might need to buy some equipment, enroll in a gym, find a friend with whom you can exercise, find a group that practices something that interests you and whose timing fits your schedule, and/or maybe convince your family to do a new activity together. During the second week, you should get used to the new routine; by the third week, you should be well on your way to establishing a vigorous exercise routine. At the end of the month, your exercise program should be in place. Don't make excuses. If you don't do it now that you have all the motivation and stamina, you will never do it!

TAKE 5

> **Learn**: Understand why and how much exercise is necessary.

> **Goal**: Follow the 32 Mondays Vigorous Exercise Program in four weeks.

> **Plan**: Decide what exercises you will do and when you will do them.

> **Monitor**: Maintain an exercise journal.

> **Reward**: Treat yourself to a new exercise outfit.

KEY POINTS

> Vigorous exercise helps you physically and psychologically.

> Twenty-five percent of weight loss is muscle, which you must regain with strength-training exercise.

> One pound (450 grams) of muscle consumes 50 to 100 calories.

> Focus primarily on muscle development and fat burning through both aerobic and anaerobic exercise.

> You need two to three days per week of a vigorous exercise program.

> Plan your vigorous exercise days and your meals accordingly.

> Forget about energy bars and drinks. Leave them to the athletes!

> Maintain your routines as much as possible.

STEP 12
FRUITS AND VEGETABLES

SUGGESTED TIME FRAME: 2 WEEKS

I am sure you have heard thousands of times about the benefits of fruits and vegetables. Sure, they are healthy, and they are what you need to eat to maintain your weight. While this is true, I am going use a different approach, just in case you are not already convinced about the need to eat many varied fruits and vegetables.

One thing all fruits and vegetables have in common is a high percentage of fiber. If you remember from **Step 8: Carbohydrates**, fiber does not carry calories but helps you increase and extend the sense of fullness. When you eat fruits and vegetables with your meals, you feel full earlier, causing you to stop eating earlier, and you won't feel the need to eat for a longer time.

Fruits and vegetables are packed with vitamins, minerals, antioxidants, and other important nutrients. Vitamins and minerals have not only enormous health benefits, but they also have energizing power, which makes you feel better and therefore more active. This helps motivate you to walk to the grocery store instead of driving there. When you feel more active, you move more and therefore you expend more energy. This is tremendously beneficial for your weight management program.

One thing fruits and vegetables don't share with each other is sugar composition. Vegetables are low in sugars, while fruits have significant quantities of sugars hidden in their fiber. This is why you need to be careful with the quantities of fruit you eat each day. One to two servings of fruit a day are enough. Remember that fruit has to be eaten at the end of a meal to avoid a huge insulin response from its sugars. Never have them by themselves as snacks, but eat them with some protein and fat to reduce the insulin spike. You should consider fruit as fat-free sweets. Be careful with fruit juices. Review **Step 3: Drinks** if you have forgotten the effect of fruit juices in your weight management program.

Because vegetables are low in sugar and calories, there is no limit on how many you can eat, with the exception of starchy vegetables like white potatoes and carrots. The more you eat, the more you'll benefit from the feeling of fullness from their fiber and from the richness of their vitamins and minerals. Remember to choose low sugar fruits and vegetables, which in most cases means those with a low glycemic index (GI) and low glycemic load (GL); these include berries, apples, pears, and oranges, and all vegetables except for potatoes, carrots, peas, and sweet potatoes.

Eating Vegetables: Making the Transition

Fruits and vegetables—especially vegetables—hold a stigma for most people, and more specifically among those who have at some time or another followed a diet, when most probably they have been asked to basically "eat vegetables."

In general, we have inaccurately been educated that vegetables are diet food, boring, and not tasty. You need to re-educate your palate, the same way you have in all the previous steps when learning to avoid highly palatable food that is rich in fat, salt, and sugar, and ready-to-eat meals, soft drinks, fast food, and sugary and salty snacks.

Vegetables are perfect to complete any pasta, rice, meat, or fish meal you want to prepare. Begin with easy ones like carrot, pumpkin, or zucchini, and then move on to the dark green, leafy ones. If you add vegetables to any stir-fry, you can be sure the result will be fantastic. There are so many different vegetables that you can change the recipes by just changing the type of vegetable, which allows you to be creative and not get bored with your meals.

Have you considered why you generally like vegetables when they are served in a restaurant? Chefs know how to prepare them to preserve all the texture and flavor. There is nothing more boring and with less taste than a bunch of vegetables that have been overboiled. All the flavors, vitamins, and minerals are left behind in the water when vegetables are abused that way.

However, it is important to be careful: sometimes you like the vegetables in the restaurants because they are cooked with plenty of fat and have other unhealthy condiments like MSG. But don't worry, once you have learned how to cook and appreciate vegetables, you will be able to detect whether a vegetable is loaded with unhealthy ingredients or it has been cooked the right way.

How to Boil Veggies the Right Way

First, you must select your vegetables and cut them to the appropriate size according to the cooking time. The longer it takes, the smaller the individual pieces should be. So cut broccoli, cauliflower, and similar vegetables in pieces the size of a fist, zucchini into one-inch chunks, and green beans and carrots into one-inch pieces.

A pressure cooker is ideal for broccoli, cauliflower, carrots, and green beans. You only need half a cup of water with a dash of salt. Cook them for about twelve minutes.

In a conventional pan, use two cups of water with salt and cover the pan. Use just enough heat to boil the water gently until the vegetables are tender, about twenty minutes.

Zucchini, spinach, kale, and similar vegetables take only two or three minutes to cook, so stir-frying is the best option for them.

How to Prepare the Perfect Vegetable Soup

You can also boil a mix of many vegetables like carrots, onions, zucchini, mushrooms, spinach, bok choy, kale, garlic, and onions. Cut the veggies into small pieces. Cook in water for about twenty minutes. You can stir-fry the veggies in some olive oil and use chicken or vegetable broth instead of water for more flavor, and use a food processor to puree if you prefer.

How to Make the Perfect Stir-Fry

This is an excellent dish to maintain all the flavor of vegetables and mix it with meat, chicken, tofu, shrimp, pork, or fish. The secret of a stir-fry is to heat the pan with olive oil until the oil starts smoking and then add the vegetables. Use a wok if you have one. The shape of the wok distributes the heat for the whole pan having more surface to "fry" the food. Always use high temperatures and stir continuously until all ingredients are golden. Add salt to taste. Salt removes the juices out of the food, and the juices will evaporate from the pan quickly because you are using a high temperature. After adding salt, reduce the heat to finish cooking the ingredients and cover to avoid evaporation.

Add broth at the end if your stir-fry is too dry or if you want a juicy dish.

Some Practical Tips to Add More Fruits and Vegetables to Your Meals

› Plan your meals ahead of time, and always include two servings a day of fruit and at least three to five of vegetables.

› Remember from **Step 4: Composition and Organization of Meals**, that every dinner should include a main vegetable, different every day. Include other vegetables during the day, like celery, carrots, or vegetable soup for a snack, a salad for lunch, tomato sauce with your pasta, etc.

› Take advantage of the sweetness of fruit, especially bananas and berries, and use it in your yogurt instead of sugar.

› Creams are easy to eat, and cauliflower cream tastes like potato. Everybody loves it.

› Have plenty of variety in your salads by using all imaginable ingredients, not just lettuce, tomatoes, and carrots. Think of celery, fennel, spinach, radishes, peppers, onions… you get the idea.

› Try to introduce a new vegetable every week.

› Consider having a green smoothie or protein shake with veggies added.

SUGGESTED TIME FRAME

You have two weeks here. You might use the first one to eat more fruits, which most people usually find easier than vegetables. Use the second week to eat any vegetables at least once a day and to get used to all the vegetable varieties in the grocery store, learn how to use them, cook them, and start to love them!

TAKE 5

› **Learn**: Understand why fruits and vegetables are important and how many you need.

› **Goal**: Include three to five servings of different vegetables and two servings of fruits daily.

› **Plan**: Decide what, when, and how you will eat your daily fruits and vegetables.

› **Monitor**: Follow your food journal.

› **Reward**: Treat yourself to a wok and a pressure cooker for your veggies.

KEY POINTS

›   Fruits and vegetables are packed with fiber, which stabilizes your metabolism.

›   Fruit has high sugar content. Limit fruits to two servings per day, and have them with other food (fat and protein) or after a meal.

›   Do not equate vegetables with dieting. They can enrich any dish with flavor!

›   There is no limit for vegetable consumption, with the exception of starchy vegetables—avoid them as much as possible.

›   Learn how to cook vegetables and add them to any dish and any meal.

STEP 13
SLEEP

SUGGESTED TIME FRAME: 1 WEEK

This is an easy step to follow. You just need to be convinced of the importance of sleep. As soon as your body becomes used to the benefits of a good and long sleep, you will need sleep to properly function, and you will start to see results: you'll feel better, more relaxed, and you will see weight loss results.

There are a few important misconceptions about sleeping. In general, adults tend to think sleeping is only necessary for kids and older people. You try to squeeze so many things in a day that you end up taking time from your seven to eight hours of sleep. You think you are okay with a few hours per night, and that you'll be back to full speed with a morning coffee. Well, the truth is you are not okay. You need enough hours to allow all the restorative processes to take place in your body. Those processes occur at night when your body is at rest with minimal activity.

The second huge misconception is that sleeping makes you fat, and therefore no sleeping makes you thinner. You think that because you are active when not asleep, you expend more calories and hence lose weight. Well, it is true you spend more calories when active compared to when asleep, but as we discussed in **Step 11: Vigorous Exercise**, it is difficult to lose weight by just exercising. Although there are lots of benefits from exercising that will help you with your weight management process, the calorie-burning itself is minimal comparing to the effort it requires.

Lack of sleep has negative effects on your weight management efforts that cannot be overcome by burning a few extra calories when you're awake.

Hormones and Sleep

Have you ever wondered why you are so hungry the day after a sleepless night?

An important hormonal process takes place at night. This process helps you control your weight and adjust the mechanism that works in your body during the day to stop the feeling of hunger. This mechanism burns calories and fat and manages cravings, which is wonderful! When you don't have enough sleep, you don't have enough of those hormones, and the whole system that stops you from being hungry and helps you burn calories fails.

The growth factor hormone (GFH), the most important hormone that helps you at night, is released during Stage 3 of your sleep cycle[38]. Therefore, the more uninterrupted sleep you have, the more GFH will be released and the more you will benefit from its positive actions over your weight management mechanisms—basically fat burning. To release the GFH, you need to have an almost-empty stomach. That's why, if you remember, I have already recommended you not eat anything right before going to bed, especially not carbohydrates which activate insulin more than any other food[39].

If you don't sleep enough hours, the secretion of leptin (the hormone that makes you feel full) will be cut short and the secretion of ghrelin (the hormone that makes you feel hungry) will increase. If you do your math, that will make you feel extra hungry the day after a night of poor or insufficient sleep. More specifically, you will crave carbohydrates, which will trigger an insulin peak.

You need seven to eight hours of uninterrupted sleep at night[40]. Not too many of us can say we achieve that, but it should be your goal. This easy step will help you maintain your weight, and the only effort you have to make is committing to go to bed at an appropriate time to allow you to sleep for seven to eight hours.

If you wake up several times at night and are overweight, consider seeing a sleep specialist. Studies have shown that night apnea is more prevalent in overweight people than in thin ones, and the problem improves dramatically with weight loss[41]. Once overweight people lose weight, they sleep better, and this helps them maintain the weight loss. See another cycle here?

Practical Ways to Get More Sleep

Unless you have a sleeping disorder, the main reason you don't get enough hours of sleep is because you go to sleep too late. You have so many commitments, and by bedtime, you still have things to do. When you are finally done, you want some time to relax, to be with your partner, call a friend, check your email, go on Facebook, watch a movie, or read a book.

To get the necessary seven to eight hours of sleep your body needs, start by fixing a bedtime based on when you have to get up, and don't forget to allow time for your bedtime routine before falling asleep. Try to reorganize your time at home with your bedtime in mind, and do not leave things to the last minute. If you are running out of time, finish the essentials and leave the other stuff for the next day or for the weekend. Remember, a lot in this program has to do with being organized, so if you got this far, you know you have to develop and maintain certain routines; sleep is no exception.

Do you have kids? Do you get onto them for going to bed too late? For leaving things to the last minute? Apply what you tell them to yourself. You have exactly the same problem. However, you are older and more experienced and should be able to change your bad habits.

SUGGESTED TIME FRAME

Only one week here—come on! You only need to accept the fact that proper sleep is tremendously important, and take your sleep time seriously.

TAKE 5

› **Learn**: Understand why you need enough sleep hours.

› **Goal**: Sleep at least seven to eight uninterrupted hours.

› **Plan**: Determine when you need to get to sleep to have seven to eight hours of sleep each night.

› **Monitor**: Write how many hours a day you sleep in your food, exercise, and sleep journal.

› **Reward**: Treat yourself to a nice new fluffy pillow.

KEY POINTS

› Growth factor hormone (GFH) is released at night after a few hours of sleep.

› You need at least seven to eight hours of uninterrupted sleep to benefit from GFH.

› Poor sleep blocks leptin, which makes you feel full, and activates ghrelin, which makes you feel hungrier.

› Proper sleep helps with weight management and with all of your body's repair and healing mechanisms.

STEP 14
GO ORGANIC

SUGGESTED TIME FRAME: 1 WEEK

You are almost done. Now you need to learn about the importance of organic foods.

The requirements for food to be considered "certified organic" are quite strict. In the United States, the United States Department of Agriculture (USDA) issues such certification, so look for the USDA Organic label in the product. In other countries, search for the specific authority regulating organic certification, and look for the labels approved for those products.

Here is a definition from Organic.com:

Simply stated, organic produce and other ingredients are grown without the use of pesticides, synthetic fertilizers, sewage sludge, genetically modified organisms, or ionizing radiation. Animals that produce meat, poultry, eggs, and dairy products do not take antibiotics or growth hormones[42].

There is a large body of evidence about the negative health effects of some of the ingredients used by the food industry: pesticides, herbicides, fungicides, preservatives, enhancers, colorants, genetically modified organisms—and the list goes on. Most conventional-food producers will argue the products they use are legal and approved by the FDA and are therefore safe. But because the human body has evolved over centuries and is designed to process a natural diet, it cannot quickly adapt to the new ingredients used in food production to improve productivity, palatability, taste, and shelf life. Many of these ingredients have a negative effect on your body's normal functioning and create disruptions that mean weight gain and illness.

Recent studies try to demonstrate organic food consumption doesn't necessarily lead to health improvement. Those studies were on the front pages of the news not too long ago[43, 44]. Don't let those studies fool you. In the same way the scientific world has been able to determine the negative effects of some products that were initially deemed safe and were eventually banned, there are dozens of products used in agriculture, livestock, and food manufacture about which you know little. For most of them, you will never know. Products are approved based on information available at the time. By the time there is enough evidence of any risk, the product is investigated, and the right conclusion is derived for regulations to be changed, the harm is already done. The lesson here is that the fewer artificial and potentially harmful products you put into your body, the better you can prevent future damage.

Allergenic Foods

More people are developing food allergies these days. In the past, an occasional person might have a food allergy, but today we see not only more kids born with or developing food allergies, but also more adults experiencing allergies at older ages. While scientists run studies to ascertain the reasons for the increase in food allergies, most of them are not conclusive, but it seems that diet and environmental factors like pollution and chemical exposure can be part of the explanation[45]. I agree with some studies that indicate that one of the most important reasons for the food allergy increase throughout our population is because we have adulterated our nutrition for the past two or three decades[46].

We constantly subject our bodies to new additives, which may in turn interact with other components and create issues that researchers find too complicated to fully understand so far. These interactions are too much for our bodies, which react the only way they can: they develop allergies to fight the foreign invaders. But we have forgotten how to listen to our bodies—or never even learned what they were saying—so we stop eating the product we think is responsible for the allergy and keep eating all the other artificial stuff. Sooner or later we will develop another allergy, which we probably won't be able to read either.

Try to eat and live as naturally and free of artificial chemicals as possible to avoid overstressing your body by making it process ingredients that are unnatural for your metabolism. This "natural" way of eating includes also eating organic as much as possible to avoid pesticides, herbicides, and other hidden ingredients. I assure you that you will see and feel the difference very soon. Your hair, skin, mood, and attitude will improve, and even your blood test results and overall health will improve without any extra effort or medications.

In 1947 in "Anytown, USA," you could read advertisements explaining all the great benefits of using a new product called DDT to kill any animal intruder and how safe it was to use at home. A few years later, the product was banned in most countries for any application, and today we can't imagine how DDT was ever used as a household insecticide. But some countries from which we import produce allow the use of products (such as DDT) that are banned in the United States, so we may be consuming those in conventional products without being aware.

Bisphenol-A (BPA) has also been used for a long time in making baby bottles and other plastics. Only recently has the general population become aware of its toxicity. And just when the general population began to understand the negative effects of BPA, we learned alternative products used for bottles can also be harmful.

These are only two examples of ingredients that are harmful to the body. Often it is the way these additives interact with one another that makes the effect especially bad. For instance, nitrates and nitrites used in processed meats are two of the worst preservatives you can consume. Together, they generate nitrosamines, which are toxic. So sometimes it is not only about the additives, but also how they may change when exposed to different conditions, other chemicals, or time.

My Journey to Organic Food

It took me a long time to be convinced about the benefits of eating organic food. At first I thought as long as I ate as healthy as possible, my body would benefit and I would be all right. I didn't realize how many unrecognized and unknown products I was ingesting in every single meal. The combination of all those artificial ingredients represented a huge impact to my health. I started to get more and more interested when my older daughter was born and I started to pay attention to how girls were "developing" at an earlier age than ever before. I realized kids have their entire lives to accumulate pesticides, added hormones, heavy metals, and other toxins. When I started to investigate the possibilities and availability of organic food (ten years ago), I found there weren't many options, and the ones available were expensive and not always of the best quality. I started buying my fruits and vegetables from local farmers, with the hope they wouldn't use many pesticides and I would at least be able to have fruits and vegetables that were as fresh as possible. I also ended up not eating chicken because I couldn't bear the idea of eating all the hormones used to raise chickens—and more specifically, of feeding them to my young children—and I was lucky enough to find a good source of organic beef.

Availability of Organic Food

Today, things are different. We have communities that have committed themselves to the pursuit of high-quality and healthy foods[47]. Thanks to advances in science that have demonstrated some of the adverse effects of the additives in our food, organic food producers have been able to defend some of their principles of providing healthy and natural products. They have raised awareness as well as demand for healthy foods such as dairy, chicken, beef, pork, most fruits and vegetables, rice, pasta, coffee, wine, and others. One of the positives of our society is that thanks to the law of supply and demand, availability of such products has been growing nonstop for the last few years. With all the potential harm around that you will probably never know about, it is better to play it safe and try to avoid the harmful products included in our foods that you have learned about as well as the potential ones like pesticides, fertilizers, herbicides, fungicides, added hormones, and artificial products.

> *Do you want to know where to buy organic? Check http://www. organicstorelocator.com/. Choose family owned organic brands when you can.*

How to Go Organic and Not Break the Bank

You will pay a price for quality food that hasn't been manipulated to increase production. If you look carefully, you will find the difference in price between organic and conventional products for some basic and essential foods is not that significant; for example lettuce, carrots, celery, bananas, and mushrooms. Of course, you need to compare organic products with high-quality conventional ones, as comparing organic foods with cheap products that can have anything in them is like comparing apples and oranges. For example, the price difference between a quality brand of conventional milk and an organic brand is not much. And there are options for finding cheaper organic products; one source is Kiplinger's "Best Places to Buy Organic Foods Without Going Broke."[48]

How to Prioritize Organics

When considering the dilemma of "to buy or not to buy" organic food, it is important to prioritize what matters to you and your family.

In my opinion, the priority should be to get rid of any external hormones. You should be alarmed that girls are reaching puberty earlier because of the hormones they ingest from the meat they eat. Thus, organic chicken and meat should be the priority. If you can't find organic, go at least for "natural"—just understand the meaning of that is quite imprecise.

From the FDA website:

"The FDA has considered the term "natural" to mean that nothing artificial or synthetic (including all color additives regardless of source) has been included in, or has been added to, a food that would not normally be expected to be in that food. However, this policy was not intended to address food production methods, such as the use of pesticides, nor did it explicitly address food processing or manufacturing methods, such as thermal technologies, pasteurization, or irradiation. The FDA also did not consider whether the term "natural" should describe any nutritional or other health benefit."[49]

Grass-fed beef is another option, although the definition of grass-fed is quite imprecise, too[50]. Not only are grass-fed meat and milk richer in omega-3 (the good fat) and lower in saturated fats (the bad fats), but if you go for cage-free chicken and eggs and pasture-fed beef, you'll also avoid eating animals that have been treated miserably, and you're more likely to avoid potential contamination with E. coli.

Wild fish equals grass-fed, and farmed fish equals conventional (they are raised using non-natural food). Farmed fish has more contaminants and antibiotics than wild fish. And according to Cleveland Clinic, "Although farmed salmon may have slightly more *omega-3 fatty acids*, it also has 20.5 percent more saturated fat content — and that's *fat you do not want.*"[51] Remember that tuna and swordfish should be eaten no more than every two weeks because of high mercury concentrations.

Next, try to select organic fruits and vegetables you eat in their entirety, like berries, cauliflower, lettuce, and greens and with the skin like apples and pears. Choose only organic grapes and celery because the conventional ones are packed with fungicides to prevent fungal infections. If your budget doesn't allow you to completely transition to organics, those that have a thick skin, like pineapple or watermelon, are less likely to be harmful. Be sure to peel all fruits and vegetables that are not organic, or at the very least wash them with one of the special solutions that might reduce some of the pesticides still on the skin.

Then, I would prioritize fruits and vegetables in which the price difference is almost non-appreciable, like bananas, lettuce, carrots, celery, potatoes, and onions. I know there will always be a price difference, but organic food is worth it. Not only does organic taste better, but from the health point of view, it's better for you if you can make the effort to pay for it.

While I always advocate choosing organic foods over conventional ones, you don't need to prioritize changing from those that are usually much more expensive than conventional ones, like asparagus, or those you don't eat very often or are not available organically grown.

If you don't have organic fruit and vegetables available, try to at least buy from a local farmer who may use fewer chemicals. Buying locally also means the food doesn't need preservatives to survive the long-distance travel and time on your supermarket's shelf. For a list of the "Dirty Dozen" and "Clean Fifteen" foods as well as other important products to buy organic, visit the Environmental Working Group's website: *www.foodnews.org*.

Manufactured/Processed Food

In the case of manufactured products like hummus, guacamole, yogurt, soup, chicken broth, and tomato sauce, organic varieties are often more difficult to find, and the prices are usually much higher than for conventional ones. It is a good idea to spend a few days investigating what is available and their prices, and always go to the organic aisle to look for special offers or sales and stock up on those. In my home, organic chicken broth and organic tomato sauce are always in the pantry. Rice and whole-grain pasta come next. If you simply cannot find organic whole-grain pasta, always choose conventional whole-grain over organic white.

If you can't afford, can't find, or are not interested in buying organic products, at least read the ingredient list to avoid artificial colors, flavors, and preservatives as much as possible. These pose similar risks to pesticides, fungicides, and other chemical products we have been talking about in this step.

By now, you have been on the 32 Mondays Weight Management Program long enough to have stopped buying processed food, and you are eating out fewer times a week. You are already saving enough money to go organic on most of the products I am recommending. Compare how much money you are saving after changing your eating habits with how much extra money you are spending by buying organic food, and I can assure you that you are still saving a good deal of money.

Highly Processed Foods

To avoid highly processed foods, the rule is simple: if the color is too exotic or unnatural, or it contains too many ingredients (including sugars) and/or the names are too complex, don't eat it. Following this rule is a simple alternative to reading long lists of ingredients in each label and will help you select the more natural products in the grocery store. Or cook food yourself or make other choices. For example, if those cupcakes with blue frosting look suspicious, go for plain whole-wheat or organic muffins, or bake them yourself at home from scratch with natural food coloring and a cream cheese-based frosting. Those hot dogs you are planning for the barbecue with friends are full of nitrites and nitrates. Invest in your health and get the organic ones or switch to organic chicken.

Unfortunately, when you constantly eat all those colorants, your body becomes overly sensitive to them. The negative effects add up year after year, and that could be the reason why one day you realize that you have developed sensitivity to lactose, gluten, or peanuts when you never had it before. I have two interesting stories about food colorants, both with my two daughters who are not used to eating colorant-rich foods.

The first is about my older daughter when she was eight. One night she had blue cotton-candy ice cream and spent the whole night vomiting. The sheets were stained blue, and although I washed them immediately, they stayed blue forever. Believe me, all those nasty products are not good for anybody, and even less so for kids, so use the rule I mentioned before: quickly spot and avoid highly processed foods.

Go Organic for Weight Management

I hope I have been able to convince you of the health benefits of going organic. I am now going to give you another benefit, in case those weren't enough.

As you've learned, appropriate weight management depends in large part on the accurate control of your metabolic functions through hormones, enzymes, and other natural metabolic constituents. Everything is in a delicate equilibrium. When you introduce external components like pesticides, antibiotics, artificial hormones, and many other contaminants found in conventional food, those with a chemical structure similar to any found in your body, such as hormone receptors, hormones, and enzymes, sometimes interact with and disrupt your body's normal functioning.

Let's remember, for example, how artificial sweeteners trick your hormonal response by sending a signal that sweet is in your bloodstream. Your body thinks that is sugar and sends the signal to remove it through insulin, but since no real sugar or calories are found, another signal will be sent to make you hungry so you'll eat and give your body real sugar.

In a similar way, certain chemical compounds called obesogens can disrupt the weight management hormonal equilibrium [52]. The fewer artificial components you add to your diet, the less you will interfere with your body's regulatory mechanisms, many of them designed to be in equilibrium and give you the right sense of hunger and fullness.

SUGGESTED TIME FRAME

This step is not difficult, complicated, or hard to maintain. However, it affects two important factors of your day-to-day life: time and budget. The results of following this step will not be seen immediately, but you will benefit in the middle to long term.

It may take some time to realize which organic foods are worth buying (how much they cost compared to conventional foods), where to find them, and how to stock them in your pantry, refrigerator, or freezer when you find a good deal. Take some time initially to master the organic sections of the grocery store, and soon you will be as efficient as you are with conventional products. Learning how to find the most beneficial products and how to impact your wallet as little as possible is totally worthwhile for your health and weight management.

It costs the same to buy a hamburger in a fast-food chain as it does to buy the organic ingredients and cook it at home. That's without considering the extra money and unhealthy trans-fat calories you would add at the restaurant when also ordering chips, beverages, and dessert. Come on, go for organic, cook it at home, and enjoy a healthy and delightful meal! And remember that money spent on health and weight improvement and illness prevention is money you won't need to spend on your future health and weight management.

TAKE 5

› **Learn**: Understand why organic food is better than conventional.

› **Goal**: Eat organic food as much as possible.

› **Plan**: Determine how to recognize and buy affordable organic products.

› **Monitor**: Look for products on sale in your preferred grocery stores.

› **Reward**: Treat yourself to a nice organic shower gel.

KEY POINTS

› By going organic, you can avoid most of the harmful components in food. Pesticides, herbicides, fungicides, hormones, food additives, and color and flavor enhancers are harmful. They disrupt metabolic equilibrium, increase risk of disease, and cause weight gain.

› You can go organic without breaking the bank by prioritizing.

› Choose organic when the difference in price is negligible.

› Choose thick-skinned fruits and vegetables if you must buy conventional.

› You can afford organic food by eating out less often and avoiding processed food.

STEP 15
BE HAPPY FOR THE REST OF YOUR LIFE

SUGGESTED TIME FRAME: 1 WEEK

Hey! Be happy! You are done!

I know. The first thing you are going to say is, "Hah! It is easy to say, as if life is so easy, and it is enough to decide to be happy and then voilà! I'll be happy."

We all have commitments, problems, families to care for, and misfortunes. Some of us may be more fortunate than others. Some of us can't simply organize or get any better at improving our lives. We get in a tunnel where everything seems dark and deep, and there seems to be no escape. The more miserable we feel, the deeper we dig into the tunnel.

There are many things that can help you move out of that tunnel, one step at a time. The 32 Mondays Weight Management Program will guide you to take one of those steps but there are many others that you might want to explore if you haven't done so. Think about spending time outdoors, especially in contact with nature. Enjoy the sight of water running down a fall, the sound of a rushing river, or the peace of a creek. Breathe the smell of flowers or trees. Observe an animal, maybe simply a squirrel or a butterfly. Really spend time in nature and your mood will improve. Your senses will become more receptive to other changes you might need to make in your life. Being outdoors will increase your vitality, which is essential when thinking about modifying your current lifestyle[53]. According to the lead author of a series of studies at the University of Rochester published in the *Journal of Environmental Psychology*, "Research has shown that people with a greater sense of vitality don't just have more energy for things they want to do, they also have more resilience to physical illnesses. One of the pathways to health may be to spend more time in natural settings."[54]

You can also explore options like meditation, yoga, listening to music, or learn a new skill like drawing or cooking. Save some time each week to play a board game with your kids, go to a concert, or find time to have a coffee with a friend. Look for those activities that may help you feel good and optimistic.

An optimistic way of thinking, living, and feeling can help you tremendously when coping with your more-or-less complicated life and misfortunes. And being optimistic is not just about seeing rainbows—it can also help you build your new project in life![55] Obviously, it can help you tremendously when trying to change things in your life—like right now when you are adopting the 32 Mondays Weight Management Program forever.

This Program will not return your health, your marriage, or your loved ones. It is not even going to bring you money, total peace, or satisfaction. But it is going to help you think and act in the right direction to be able to cope and manage your weight in the best possible way. By improving something so important as your relationship with food, exercise, and sleep while getting in control of your weight, you will feel much more empowered and ready to manage appropriately the rest of the things that matter in your life.

Be happy, and don't feel miserable for getting rid of the food you loved in your past life. We've already talked a lot about health and the importance of changing those bad habits and learning new ones. We've discussed how to re-educate your way of nourishing your body and the way to enjoy your food. By now, you should be done with that negative thinking and you should have moved to positive thinking where you shouldn't feel like you are missing anything. The only thing you are losing is weight, which you shouldn't be missing at all!

Adopt an Addiction to Positivity

If your body is well-fed and your hormones are in balance, if you are sleeping well and exercising, chances are you will feel energetic, optimistic, and happy. That, coupled with looking better, should give you a more positive outlook and a rewarding life.

In the same way that sugar, salt, and bad foods are addictive, so are exercising, eating well, and being happy. So, let's develop these "positive addictions."

Remember, willpower is limited. The more you have planned and organized ahead of time, the less energy you will need to make decisions about what and when to eat. Have next week's meal plans ready by the end of this weekend, and have all the ingredients you need ready to make the menu plan happen. Always have the right ingredients available for snacks and emergencies.

The Candy Bar: How to Be Happy Practically

Do you feel miserable because you are dreaming about having a candy bar? Or maybe you feel guilty and miserable because you already had one in the middle of your day or right before going to bed. Whatever the situation, your basic dilemma is that a candy bar is making you feel miserable, whether because you wish you could eat one or because you feel guilty because you just ate it.

Stop feeling miserable. Have your candy bar, but please, enjoy it! Feel and enjoy every bit of it. Be happy! Let your endorphins run through your body, and give thanks to whomever you believe in and relax. Don't feel guilty—be proactive. Rather than beating yourself up for a failure, plan the right meal for tonight or tomorrow.

If you try to apply the candy bar example to most of the things happening in your life, you will feel better. You can't always be fighting against natural desires and getting mad every time things don't go the way you expected. You have to create a natural flow. Let things happen. Most of the time there is a reason for what is making you unhappy, uncomfortable, or unbalanced, and if you analyze it, you can find that reason. Even if you don't find the reason, avoid the fight and the resulting tiredness and impotence of not getting things the way you expected. Be more flexible and relaxed with your menus during the weekend to start the new week fresh as a way to ease back into your healthy lifestyle.

The Importance of Positive Visualization

This might sound silly, but instead of being mad because you are not eating burgers for lunch anymore, visualize the fat leaving your belly, see the new you, and substitute a nice chicken salad for that burger. If you missed the bus, don't get mad: walk for a few blocks to get your exercise. You lost fifty dollars on the street? Tell yourself that maybe someone who really needed the money found it. Your kid is sick today? Maybe you needed more quality time together. Try to find a way to turn whatever is happening that is difficult to cope with or making you feel bad or negative into something more positive. Try to transform that experience into one that makes you feel better and helps you move on to something else that is more positive.

TAKE 5

> **Learn**: Understand how being happy helps your health and weight management.

> **Goal**: Maintain a positive attitude most of the time to help you be happy.

> **Plan**: Always look at the positives in any situation.

> **Monitor**: Pay attention to how many times a day you get mad and how many you could have avoided.

›   **Reward**: Treat yourself to a smiley-face pendant or keychain to carry with you.

KEY POINTS

›   A positive attitude can help you cope with anything going on in your life.

›   Trade your bad food addiction for exercise and good nutrition addictions.

›   Happiness can also be addictive.

›   Have the occasional candy bar without feeling miserable.

›   Practice positive visualization to make healthy eating choices.

›   Let things happen in your life without fighting them.

Accept, analyze, and move on!

PART III

ADDITIONAL INFORMATION

There are still three more aspects I would like to cover that I consider important for healthy living and weight management. Since they are not applicable to everybody I have left them for the end. They are: Kids and Healthy Eating, Supplements, and Pharmaceuticals.

Kids and Healthy Eating

Nothing hurts me more than seeing overweight kids. Believe me, the suffering they experience (or are about to experience if they are still too young to be aware) is overwhelming. Not only do they suffer peer discrimination—bullying—but they also suffer a lack of self-esteem and an unhealthy problem they most likely will carry with them for the rest of their lives.

Many parents blame inherited slow metabolism or children's food preferences, when most of the time it is just a matter of education on how to eat. I wonder why parents go to so much trouble and sacrifice to get the best education for their kids, bring them to the best schools, make them earn the best grades, and push them into lots of after-school activities, but they don't think about how to educate their kids about healthy eating. I know it is hard, but I wonder if it is harder than helping them learn multiplication or equations.

Teaching your kids good nutrition habits and how to buy and prepare the healthiest ingredients are lessons in life as important as any other, and they will last forever. You might forget how to solve an equation, but you will never forget what a healthy lifestyle is if you have learned it.

Parental Influence

I was sad to learn about the death of a woman who worked for my husband. She was loved by everybody in the company. She was only forty-nine years old, but she was quite overweight. While there might have been some inherited metabolic abnormality (her mother was also overweight, and she also died in her forties), her nutrition habits weren't healthy and she didn't exercise. I am pretty sure her mother shared the same eating and exercising habits, so that's what she taught her daughter because she didn't know better. The sad result is this woman had been medicated for a long time for high blood pressure, diabetes, and heart disease, and she ended up facing a sudden death at a young age, probably as a result of her overweight problem and its associated complications. We moms love our kids immensely, and we try to do our best to raise them healthy and happy, so I have to assume this woman's mother didn't know enough about nutrition to feed her daughter more appropriately.

You have this book in your hands, so you already know better. You have the ability to teach your kids exactly the same things you have learned for yourself. What works for you will work for them. You may need to skip some of the technical explanation and adapt the necessary parts to their level of comprehension, but please, don't underestimate the ability of your children to understand what is going on. Never tell them "because I say so" when they ask you why. They need to understand the reasons for the things they are being taught.

Getting Your Kids to Eat Healthy

If they are very young, almost babies, it won't take you any effort. Changing their eating habits will even simplify your life because you won't have to prepare different meals for your kids. They will grow up enjoying fruits, vegetables, nuts, quinoa, bulgur, whole-grain bread, kefir, and tofu. You might encounter some challenges when they get older and start experiencing peer pressure at school, as they probably will be eating differently than the majority. Some of their friends will think your kid's food is "yucky"; some won't even try it. But your kids will be learning self-confidence when they tell their friends how delicious their food tastes and how healthy and strong it makes them feel.

If your kids are not babies anymore but you still have some power over them, you'll have to fight a little bit to change their habits. You have probably educated them to eat food that is marketed for children, where everything healthy is camouflaged in lots of butter, bread, or pasta. Even if you spend half of your time in the kitchen developing your creativity to convince your kid to eat a single green bean (which appears as a big smile of a rice snowman's face), the moment your kids want to make their own choices (which will include food), you don't have much power anymore to decide what they eat. They need to understand what is behind the importance of good eating habits, proper sleep, and adequate exercise, and learn the meaning and effects of hypertension, high cholesterol, heart problems, and diabetes as well as the other effects of bad eating habits and being overweight. Once they understand there is a reason behind your interest in feeding them proper food, they will be ready to listen and change their attitudes.

And by the way, when you eat at a restaurant, please don't feed your kids from the kids' menu. I know it is easier and cheaper, but let them learn from the experience of trying new food. Expose them to a variety of food available in different ethnic and local restaurants.

If your kids are already teenagers, don't even try. Give them this book, cross your fingers, and hope they will listen to you for one time and read it. If it doesn't work, let's hope someday they will change their attitude. It is my plan to one day write a nutritional book addressed to teenagers.

Following are some suggestions to help you properly educate your children about nutrition and make sure they are well-nourished throughout the day.

Kids and Breakfast

All families are rushed in the morning. Whether you have one child or four, whether both parents work or one is a homemaker, in the end, you all end up rushing in the morning and making the easy decision of skipping breakfast or having quick, easy, and fight-free sugary breakfast cereals, a sugary muffin, or cookies.

If you send your kids to school with a sugary breakfast and a sandwich for lunch and then expect them to do well at school, think again. Instead you must provide them with a breakfast comprised of slow sugars, meaning complex carbs like whole wheat, brown rice, and corn, and protein and fats that can feed their brains and muscles for hours.

Your child's brain, when active, requires a large and constant supply of energy in the form of glucose. This is the reason why they need food rich in complex carbs, protein, and fats (instead of fast, simple sugars) that are slowly released and can last for hours. If you expect that brain to work for as many as six to seven hours in a row, you need to feed it properly. For a kid who maybe has walked or biked to school (if lucky) and then has gone through an hour of physical education and/or thirty minutes of playing and running at the playground, eating healthy food will help him or her stay healthy, learn more, and misbehave less.

Kids, Lunch, and Snacks

Many kids are sent to school with a sandwich and a milk or juice box for lunch. Just think how you feel by midafternoon when you are hungry (starving!), and your bad temper starts to flourish. Now imagine your kids at school after working their brains plus running with their friends. You could not realistically expect them to behave properly after a small lunch. You should provide them with the same sort of lunch you have, plus more if they are still hungry, as well as a box of milk.

It is especially important to provide kids with two snacks (morning and afternoon), as they don't have the ability to eat enough in each meal to maintain them until the next meal. These snacks should be comprised of healthy calories (cheese and fruit, some nuts, hummus with celery or carrots, or some ham with whole-wheat pretzels) and maybe a trans fat-free cookie or a small piece of quality chocolate (high in cocoa and lower in sugar). You need to consider that children are growing constantly, and some are extra active, which means they need those snacks to maintain their energy levels and have enough energy to feed their brains.

Kids and Dinner

Dinner is the meal of the day where you probably have more room to play with what you feed your kids. Hopefully you won't be in a hurry like in the morning, and you don't need to figure out something that they can easily bring to school.

Use dinner to feed your kids all the vitamins and minerals (in the form of fruits and vegetables) they might have missed during the day. Add some easy-to-digest lean protein to feed their growing muscles—especially fish, which is probably the only time of the day you can give it to your kids.

Regarding carbs: avoid them as much as possible if your kid has tendency to gain weight, and use the "brown" version (whole-grain bread, pasta, and brown rice).

Supplements

This is my point of view: if you eat properly, you shouldn't need many supplements. Having said this, we need to determine what it means to eat properly. Well, you need to eat a variety of fruit, vegetables, and dairy products daily; red meat two times per week; and fish two or three times per week (only once per week for salmon, once every two weeks for tuna or swordfish, and other fish once or twice per week). If you also eat brown rice or other cereal, whole-wheat pasta, and whole-grain bread, and you add some seeds and olive oil, chances are you won't have any deficiencies. If you suspect you could have a deficiency because you are not eating all the basic food groups mentioned in this book, and you experience symptoms like feeling tired, or you have frequent colds or get sick often, please see your doctor before you start taking any supplements. For instance, lack of red meat can lead to an iron deficiency; lack of eggs and fish high in omegas can result in omega-3 deficiency, lack of sunlight can lead to vitamin D deficiency. If you never eat brown rice, pasta, cereal, or whole-wheat bread, you may be missing fiber and some essential minerals.

Tests are expensive, but supplements are, too. If you are taking supplements and you don't need them, you are wasting your money. Plus, if you don't know what is going on in your body, you won't know when to stop taking them. On the other hand, if you test positive for any deficiency, you can always try to fix it in a natural way by eating food rich in your deficient nutrient, and then go for a supplement if that doesn't work. (Supplements are always much more difficult to absorb than their natural equivalents.)

I only recommend three supplements for the average population:

1. Omega-3, which has *many* healthy benefits—and can help you lose weight. Fish oil is especially recommended for those who don't like to eat fish.

2. Vitamin D is recommended in winter, especially for people living in cold areas where there is not enough sun exposure to synthesize vitamin D naturally. Vitamin D-fortified milk is beneficial for everyone.

3. Calcium supplements are suggested for teenagers and women in menopause because of the high dose of calcium required at those stages of life, as well as for anyone not consuming enough dairy to cover their calcium needs. Plant-based calcium like collard greens, broccoli, and tofu or soybeans add some quantity, but sometimes it is quite difficult to get the total amount you need. See the chart at *http://nof.org/calcium* for a list of calcium-rich foods.

Some doctors and researchers don't believe that calcium supplements are the most effective way to get the calcium you need, or even that calcium supplementation is effective[56]. Decide with your doctor whether you should take them or not. Some forms of calcium are more absorbable than others, and too much can be harmful[57]. You need magnesium and vitamin D to make sure you absorb it, so choose a brand that also contains those two ingredients.

Go for a brand that offers high-quality products that are purified and has the USP (United States Pharmacopeta) symbol.[58]

Remember that supplements are not a substitution for eating the proper food. Be wary of an excess of supplements, as they can be seriously harmful[59].

Some fortified products might be beneficial even if you don't have any specific deficiencies. Examples are calcium-fortified orange juice for kids and women; vitamin D-fortified milk for everyone; and fish oil for those who dislike fish. It is never a bad idea to buy a fortified product (preferably organic). Remember, the extra dollars you are investing in healthier food will be saved in health and weight improvement in the long run.

Pharmaceuticals

Your body views drugs as artificial products. They help your body manage whatever is not working properly, but they also unintentionally interact with other parts of your metabolism. Unfortunately, we live in a society that tends to overprescribe pharmaceuticals as a safety measure, so make sure you really need whatever drugs you take.

Prescription drugs also affect parts of your metabolism that can interact with your weight management. If you take pharmaceuticals to treat diabetes, high cholesterol, or hypertension, which are conditions affected by your nutrition, it is especially important to change your eating habits.

When you start to eat more naturally by avoiding highly processed foods that are packed with preservatives, colorants, trans fats, sugars, and salt, and you start eating a diet rich in fruits and vegetables, and organic as much as possible, you will see an important health improvement. Many serious (and some not so serious) conditions can be improved by better nutrition. Ask your doctor what you can do nutritionally to better manage your medical condition, and ask him or her to do periodic checks to monitor your improvement, and also to reduce your medication if possible.

You will be surprised at how much you can improve your health by changing your nutritional habits.

ACKNOWLEDGMENTS

I have to thank three people for inspiring me to write this book; the triggers who made this book alive are Jorge Luis Borges, Steve Jobs, and my beloved husband, Sergio.

The summer before my young daughter became a "lunch kid"—meaning she stayed at school for lunch and didn't come home until 3:00 p.m.—and allowed me some more time to work, I listened to the radio and heard a quote from Jorge Luis Borges, who is a twentieth-century writer, thinker, and critic. He was born in Argentina (like my husband) and lived in Spain (my country of origin) for some time, so I felt a special connection with him. He once said he needed to write in order to get the ideas out of his head and avoid going crazy by them pushing on his brain. I enjoyed the quote immensely, and I realized I had that similar need. After so many years studying, reading, thinking, observing, and analyzing all the factors involved in weight management, I had so much information and so many ideas circulating in my head that I needed to let them go. As soon as I had some time for myself, usually when running or swimming, new ideas about how to help others work on their weight management would come into my mind. So I discovered that writing a book could be the way to free my mind.

The following month, when Steve Jobs, cofounder of Apple, Inc., announced he was retiring as president, there was a trailer on CNN from Steve Jobs' commencement speech to Stanford University in 2005. He talked about how life is short and how every day is so precious, and he urged all those young people not to waste any more time and to have the courage to follow their intuition, passion, feelings, guts, or whatever they have inside. This was my second inspiration. My inner passion has always been to dedicate my time and energy to helping other people who struggle with weight management.

Unfortunately, Steve Jobs died a few months later. I wrote this acknowledgment the day after he died, and I would like to offer him a tribute, especially for the encouragement he left for us. I urge you to see that video if you ever have the opportunity to do so: *2005 Commencement Address at Stanford University. http://news.stanford.edu/news/2005/june15/jobs-061505.html.* It can be an inspiration for the trip you have ahead, too.

A few days after listening to Jobs's speech, I explained to my husband my idea of following my inspiration to write a book about weight management. He was wholly supportive and gave me the last push I needed to start writing on the first day my young daughter became a "lunch kid." Thank you, Sergio. This book is my second passion after you! I would never have started it without your unconditional support. As Julia Child's husband, Paul, said to her in the movie *Julie and Julia*, "You are the butter to my bread, the bread to my life."

APPENDIX A
RECOMMENDED RESOURCES

General reading

Kessler, David A. The End of Overeating: Taking Control of the Insatiable American Appetite. Emmaus, PA: Rodale, 2009.

McCaffrey, Dee. The Science of Skinny: Start Understanding Your Body's Chemistry and Stop Dieting Forever. Boston, MA: Da Capo Lifelong, 2012.

Miller, Janette Brand, Kaye Foster-Powell, and Fiona Atkinson. The Shopper's Guide to GI Values: The Authoritative Source of Glycemic Index Values for More than 1,200 Foods.

Moss, Michael. Salt, Sugar, Fat: How the Food Giants Hooked Us. New York: Random House, 2013.

Pollan, Michael. In Defense of Food: An Eater's Manifesto. New York: Penguin Press, 2008.

Siler, Brooke. The Pilates Body.

Videos

Soul Food Junkies

http://greencommunityconnections.org/soul-food-junkies/

Fast Food, Fat Profits

https://www.youtube.com/watch?v=slwgXXVXM3I

Active Exercise

Calories burned in 30 minutes of exercise

http://www.health.harvard.edu/diet-and-weight-loss/
calories-burned-in-30-minutes-of-leisure-and-routine-activities

Strength Training

Mayo Clinic: Strength Training Videos

http://www.mayoclinic.org/healthy-lifestyle/fitness/in-depth/strength-training/
art-20046031

Cooking and Eating Well

www.cookinglight.com

www.eatingwell.com

Fish Consumption Advisory

www.epa.gov/ost/fish

Local Harvest

www.localharvest.org

Meditation

The Meditation Society of America

www.meditationsociety.com

Sleep

The National Sleep Foundation

www.SleepFoundation.org

APPENDIX B
HEIGHT / WEIGHT / BMI CHART AND WAIST CIRCUMFERENCE VALUES[60]

Here is the way the IDF recommends measuring your waist circumference: measure in a horizontal plane, midway between the inferior margin of the ribs and the superior border of the iliac crest. (The iliac crest is the thick curved upper border of the ilium, the most prominent bone on the pelvis. You can feel the iliac crest by pushing your hands on your sides at your waist, feeling for the bone and following it down and to the front.) Once you have measured your waist circumference, compare it with the table below.

BMI	18.9 or Lower	19.0-24.9	25.0-29.9	30 or Higher
	Underweight	Healthy	Overweight	Obese

Height (in.)	Less than	Body Weight (lb.)		More than
58	90	91-118	119-142	143
59	93	94-123	124-147	148
60	96	97-127	128-152	153

61	99	100-131	132-157	158
62	103	104-135	136-163	164
63	106	107-140	141-168	169
64	109	110-144	145-173	174
65	113	114-149	150-179	180
66	117	118-154	155-185	186
67	120	121-157	158-190	191
68	124	125-163	164-197	198
69	127	128-168	169-202	203
70	131	132-173	174-208	209
71	135	136-178	179-214	215
72	139	140-183	184-220	221
73	143	144-188	189-226	227
74	147	148-193	194-232	233
75	151	152-199	200-239	240
76	155	156-204	205-245	246

Waist Circumference[61]

If your waist circumference value is larger than the following, and you have two or more of the four risk factors (high triglycerides, reduced HDL cholesterol, elevated blood pressure, or elevated fasting blood glucose), you are at risk for adult metabolic syndrome according to the IDF:

Country/Ethnic group		Waist circumference
Europids	Male	> 94 cm (37 in.)
In the USA, the ATP III values (102 cm male; 88 cm female)	Female	> 80 cm (31.5 in.)

South Asians	Male	> 90 cm (35.4 in.)
Based on a Chinese, Malay and Asian-Indian population	Female	> 80 cm
Chinese	Male	> 90 cm
	Female	> 80 cm
Japanese	Male	> 90 cm
	Female	> 80 cm
Ethnic South and Central Americans	*Use South Asian recommendations until more specific data are available*	
Sub-Saharan Africans	*Use European data until more specific data are available*	
Eastern Mediterranean and Middle East (Arab) populations	*Use European data until more specific data are available*	

APPENDIX C
CALORIES BURNED WHEN EXERCISING

Following is a list of types of exercises and the calories burned after an hour. The calculation is based in a person whose weight is around 155 pounds (70 kg) and another of 185 pounds (84 kg). Please remember that the more you weigh, the more calories you burn (it takes more energy moving a heavier mass).

The idea of this list is not to help you to calculate how many hours of exercise you need to burn the doughnut you are dreaming of. In the first place, you shouldn't eat that doughnut full of calories, sugar, and trans fats anyway. In the second place, the objective for changing your lifestyle and exercising more is to burn the extra weight you've accumulated over the years and earn a healthier body. After losing the extra weight, exercise will help you to maintain your desired weight, feel better, and live healthier.

If you pay close attention, you will realize that it takes too much exercise to burn that doughnut. You will probably never fully burn it! So don't even try to lose weigh only by exercising. You will kill yourself, and you won't succeed.

The idea of offering this list is to give you an idea of which types of exercise burn more calories. Also, it should help you realize that vacuuming is not really a calorie-burning exercise, although any type of movement is better than just sitting around.

Finally, remember that your interest in exercise is not only for calorie burning but also for muscle development; remember that muscle is a bigger calorie burner than fat tissue. Post-exercise secretion of many hormones also helps to regulate your metabolism and keep your weight management under control.

I have listed a few of the most common exercises. Go to the original source from Harvard Medical School to get the calories burned for thirty minutes of the exercise that interests you.[62]

Calories Burned in Thirty Minutes for People of Three Different Weights

Gym Activities	125 lb (57 Kg)	155 lb (70 Kg)	185 lb (84 Kg)
Aerobics, low impact	165	205	244
Cycling, mountain bike	255	316	377
Cycling, medium	240	298	355
Weight lifting, vigorous	180	223	266
Stretching, Hatha Yoga	120	149	178
Aerobics: water	120	149	178
Running, medium	240	298	355
Walking moderate	135	167	200
Swimming laps, general	300	372	444

APPENDIX D
LIST OF SUGAR NAMES[63]

- › agave nectar
- › barley malt
- › beet sugar
- › blackstrap molasses
- › brown sugar
- › buttered syrup
- › cane crystals
- › cane juice crystals
- › cane sugar
- › caramel
- › carob syrup
- › castor sugar
- › confectioner's sugar

> corn syrup

> corn sweetener

> corn syrup solids

> crystalline fructose

> date sugar

> demerara sugar

> dextrin

> dextran

> dextrose

> diastatic malt

> diastase

> d-mannose

> evaporated cane juice

> ethyl maltol

> florida crystals

> free flowing

> fructose

> fruit juice

> fruit juice concentrate

> galactose

> glucose

> glucose solids

- golden sugar
- golden syrup
- granulated sugar
- grape sugar
- grape juice concentrate
- hfcs
- high-fructose corn syrup
- honey
- icing sugar
- invert sugar
- lactose
- malt syrup
- maltodextrin
- maltose
- mannitol
- maple syrup
- molasses
- muscovado sugar
- organic raw sugar
- panocha
- powdered sugar
- raw sugar

> refiner's syrup

> rice syrup

> sorbitol

> sorghum syrup

> sucrose

> sugar

> syrup syrup

> table sugar

> treacle

> turbinado sugar

> yellow sugar

APPENDIX E
GROCERY STORE SHOPPING LIST

Remember that it is essential to maintain your serving sizes (review Step 1 if necessary) and buy organic whenever possible.

Vegetables 1 (essential items that you need to have at all times)

› lettuce or mixed greens (organic)

› baby carrots ready to eat (organic)

› celery (organic)

› onions (organic)

› garlic

Vegetables 2 (one for each day of the week)

› baby spinach (organic)

› broccoli (organic)

› cauliflower (organic)

› zucchini (organic)

> green beans

> brussels sprouts

> any other green

Other Vegetables

> potatoes (organic)

> corn

> pumpkin

> asparagus

Fruits

> oranges (organic)

> apples (organic)

> pears (organic)

> grapes (organic)

> strawberries (organic)

> blueberries (organic)

> peaches (organic)

> nectarines (organic)

> prunes (organic)

> pineapple

> watermelon

> melon

› mangoes

› avocado

Dairy (organic, fat-free, or low fat)

› milk

› yogurt or Greek yogurt (your preference)

› kefir

› cheese

› ice cream (look for a brand with a low sugar content per serving)

Meat (grass-fed, organic, or at least hormone-free) and wild fish

› ham and bacon (*must* be organic and free of nitrites and nitrates)

› poultry

› beef

› sausages

› hot dogs (*must* be organic and free of nitrites and nitrates)

› fish (wild caught, not farmed)

› eggs

Other Fresh Foods (natural, organic)

› hummus

› dips with yogurt and vegetables and no canola oil

› sauces (tomato, pesto, and others with olive oil)

› olive oil (cold-pressed, extra-virgin)

> tofu

Carbohydrates (whole-grain/whole-wheat, at least 3 grams of fiber per serving)

> breads

> pasta

> rice

> couscous

> quinoa

> bulgur

> farro

> crackers with no hydrogenated fats and no canola oil

> whole-wheat tortillas

> cereals (brown rice, kamuk, granola; no sugar added)

Treats

> dark chocolate (the darker the better)

> muffin mix (whole-wheat/whole-grain)

> brownies mix (organic)

> cookies (whole-wheat/whole-grain, organic, no trans fats)

Pizza

> Whole-wheat base to make it yourself

APPENDIX F
WEEKLY MEAL PLAN

This is an example of a meal plan for a week. As I explained in **Principle 6, Navigating the Kitchen**, you can play with the main ingredients to create different meal plans. You can also adapt your favorite meals by using whole grains, lowering fat and sugars, and increasing vegetables to fit into your weekly plan.

The idea of a meal plan is to balance the nutritional values each day. For example, if you are having a rich macaroni pasta with cheese and meat for lunch, you would need only vegetables and an egg for dinner. If that is not enough to fill you, eat some fruit with cheese, or snack and complement dinner with a Greek yogurt. Or if you know you are having cake at night to celebrate your son's birthday, have a light dinner with no other carb.

Although you will see three snacks listed for each day, only a maximum of two snacks a day is allowed. You should organize them according to your needs.

All serving sizes are single-serving unless otherwise noted.

MONDAY

Breakfast

›   whole-wheat toast with olive oil and prosciutto

›   cheese

›   coffee or tea

Snack (if more than three to four hours remain before lunch)

›   nuts

›   fruit (½ serving)

Lunch

›   tomato salad

›   macaroni with meat, tomato, and grated cheese

›   fruit

Snack (if more than three to four hours remain before dinner)

›   cheese

›   whole-grain bread

Dinner

›   steamed broccoli

›   ham omelet

›   whole-grain bread

›   fruit

›   treat

Snack (if more than three to four hours remain before bed)

> carrots with hummus

TUESDAY

Breakfast

> plain yogurt with fresh fruit

> low-sugar, high-fiber cereal

> coffee or tea

Snack (if more than three to four hours remain before lunch)

> whole-grain bread

> cheese

Lunch

> chicken with mushrooms and quinoa

> fruit

Snack (if more than three to four hours remain before dinner)

> nuts

Dinner

> vegetable cream

> bread

> ham

> ›   kefir with berries

> ›   treat

Snack (if more than three to four hours remain before bed)

> ›   carrots with hummus

WEDNESDAY

Breakfast

> ›   whole-wheat toast with tomato and ham

> ›   cheese

> ›   coffee or tea

Snack (if more than three to four hours remain before lunch)

> ›   nuts

Lunch

> ›   Surprise me! vegetable soup with lentils, bulgur, quinoa, or similar

> ›   fruit

Snack (if more than three to four hours remain before dinner)

> ›   low-fat cheese

> ›   fruit

Dinner

> ›   tomato and mozzarella salad

> › grilled salmon

> › yogurt

> › treat

Snack (if more than three to four hours remain before bed)

> › celery with guacamole

THURSDAY

Breakfast

> › whole-wheat toast with olive oil and salami

> › yogurt

Snack (if more than three to four hours remain before lunch)

> › carrots with hummus

Lunch

> › whole-wheat pasta salad with vegetables, tuna, and beans

> › yogurt with fruit

Snack (if more than three to four hours remain before dinner)

> › nuts

Dinner

> › boiled green beans with carrots and onion

> › eggs

- › fruit

- › treat

Snack (if more than three to four hours remain before going to bed)

- › mozzarella stick

- › small piece of prosciutto

FRIDAY

Breakfast

- › whole-wheat toast with cheese spread and jam

Snack (if more than three to four hours remain before lunch)

- › cheese

Lunch

- › healthy hamburger with vegetables

- › fruit

Snack (if more than three to four hours remain before dinner)

- › yogurt and fruit

Dinner

- › green salad

- › fish

› flan

Snack (if more than three to four hours remain before going to bed)

› yogurt

SATURDAY

Breakfast

› kefir

› high-fiber cereal (no sugar added or low-sugar)

Snack (if more than three to four hours remain before lunch)

› carrots with hummus

Lunch

› beef with vegetables

› fruit

Snack (if more than three to four hours remain before dinner)

› yogurt and fruit

Dinner

› green salad with egg, tuna, and nuts

› puff-pastry cake with lots of fruit

Snack (if more than three to four hours remain before going to bed)

› mozzarella stick

SUNDAY

Breakfast

› whole-wheat pancakes with a bit of butter and a bit of maple syrup

Snack (if there are more than three to four hours before lunch)

› cheese

Lunch

› stir-fry chicken and vegetables and quinoa or couscous

› fruit

Snack (if more than three to four hours remain before dinner)

› yogurt

Dinner

› green salad

› grilled fish

› yogurt

› treat

Snack (if more than three to four hours remain before going to bed)

› celery and hummus

APPENDIX G
FOOD JOURNAL TEMPLATE

WEEK	MONDAY	TUESDAY	WEDNESDAY	THURSDAY	FRIDAY	SATURDAY	SUNDAY
BREAKFAST Time:							
MORNING SNACK Time:							

LUNCH							
Time:							
AFTERNOON SNACK							
Time:							
DINNER							
Time:							
NIGHT SNACK							
Time:							

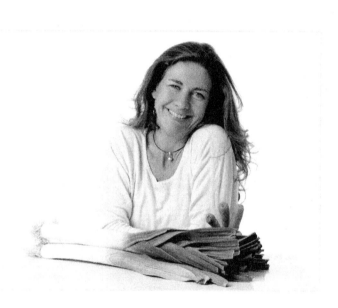

ABOUT THE AUTHOR

Arantxa Mateo is a trained biologist, nutrition specialist, and weight management mentor. Born and raised in Barcelona, Spain, Arantxa was overweight as a child, but as a teenager, she discovered she could take control of what and when to eat. That's when she decided to study biology to learn as much as possible about the science of life and its relation to nutrition and weight management.

Arantxa's personal struggles combined with her education in biology and nutrition eventually lead her to develop the 32 Mondays Weight Management Program, which is not a diet but rather an educational program to teach people how to manage their weight for the rest of their lives. Today, Arantxa no longer hides her body, and she feels in perfect harmony with herself. She is fluent in both Spanish and English, and she's excited to help others establish a new routine through her innovative program that will keep them focused on losing weight until they reach their goals. As someone who knows what it is like to struggle with healthy eating, Arantxa believes that "Food is a pleasure. Nobody deserves to be on a diet!"

Apart from the *32 Mondays online course,* which guides you through the whole program, Arantxa also offers free practical tips around weight loss and weight management, one-on-one consultations, workshops, and webinars. To find out more, visit her website, *www.32Mondays.com.*

Follow Arantxa on Facebook *https://www.facebook.com/32-Mondays-Weight-Loss-Management* or get in touch with her via email at *arantxamateo@32mondays.com.*

INDEX

A

abdominal fat 25,27, 72,73, 151, 167,170
addiction 9,29, 51-56, 71,101-103,109, 148,150
additives 47, 117, 198-206
aging 72,73, 172-174, 259, 261
artificial coloring and flavoring 106,110,203
artificial sweeteners 68, 86, 101-107, 149-155, 205
alcohol 82, 125, 167-170, 260,261
appetite 36, 61, 70, 72, 104, 152, 172, 173, 225

B

beans 48, 61-63, 85, 112, 119, 148, 158, 189, 220, 238, 245
behavior 60, 62, 81, 176
berries 42, 103, 113-120, 153, 154, 188, 190, 202, 238,244
beverages. See drinks
blood sugar 16, 61, 65, 86, 114, 131
body fat 27, 58, 68, 176, 182
body mass index (BMI) 25-30, 227
brain 12-20, 40, 51, 58-64, 70, 87, 103, 107, 115, 130, 163, 179, 218, 219
breakfast 53, 55, 71, 78, 85, 86, 106, 112, 182, 218, 242

C

cancer 27, 103, 140, 152, 159, 172
canola oil 47, 117, 239-240
carbohydrates 3,4,13, 20, 48, 49, 58-65, 69-73, 106, 112-127, 133-137, 157-161, 186-194, 240
cardiovascular disease. See heart disease 141

cheese 42-54, 84-87, 112-126, 132-150, 165, 204, 218, 239-248
chicken 2, 40-43, 46-50, 84, 113-119, 133, 143-146, 190, 200-204, 212, 242-243
chocolate 22, 40, 48-55, 64, 78, 84, 103, 107, 113, 120, 124, 133, 153, 219
cholesterol 9, 69, 75, 113, 116, 138-142, 167, 217, 221, 228
coffee 2, 32, 55, 86, 106-110, 115-118, 150-154, 174, 201, 210, 242
composition of meals 82, 111-127, 190
cooking skills 45
cortisol 72-74, 92, 184
cravings 53, 61, 86, 103, 104, 109-110, 119, 152, 194

D
dairy products 50, 146, 197
diabetes 16, 25, 27, 30, 60-65, 75, 172, 216, 217, 221
drinks 64, 68, 82, 101-110, 113, 125, 130-133, 147, 149-152, 167-170, 178, 186, 188

E
eating out 29, 122, 204, 207
eggs 50, 116, 120, 124, 197, 202, 220, 239, 245

F
fiber 58, 61-65, 85, 105, 110, 117, 131, 149-153, 157-162, 186-188
fish oil supplements 142, 220, 221
food diary 85-89, 110, 168, 170
food industry 31-37, 51, 54, 56, 138, 140, 150, 197
food labels 34, 88, 162
fruit juices 104, 105, 117, 148-153, 188

G
genetically modified organisms (GMOs) 144, 151
ghrelin 47, 71-74, 133, 179, 196
glucose 22, 52, 57-65, 70, 73, 75, 104, 109, 129-131, 149-179, 218, 234
gluten 204
glycemic index (GI) 61-63, 88-89, 117, 133, 158, 159-188
glycemic load (GL) 62-63, 88-89, 159-159, 188
granola 117-118, 240
grains 58, 61, 112, 117-119, 132, 158-162
grass-fed 202
grocery shopping 39-43
grocery store 16, 31, 36-43, 93, 106, 113, 117-121, 145, 187, 191, 204-206, 237

H

habits 5, 6, 14, 16, 31-37, 47, 52-56, 64-67, 77-81, 91-94, 101, 115, 123, 145, 148, 184, 195, 204, 210, 216, 217, 221

happy 21, 53, 91, 171, 209-213, 216

health benefits 117, 141, 163, 167, 172, 216

heart disease 140, 141, 163, 167, 172, 216

high-fructose corn syrup (HFCS) 113, 150-155, 235

hormones 3, 33, 52, 65, 67-73, 102, 106, 115, 120, 138, 148, 172, 178, 182, 194, 197, 200-206, 211, 232

hummus 84-86, 134, 203, 341-249

hydration 106, 108

hydrogenated fats 47

I

inflammation 141, 142

insulin resistance 29, 60, 64, 65, 76

International Diabetes Federation (IDF) 25-28, 76, 228

kitchen 21, 36, 43, 45-49, 108, 145, 151, 217

legumes 48, 84

leptin 70-74, 130, 150, 151, 194, 196

lifestyle 92-95, 98, 168, 171, 177, 210, 212, 216, 231

M

meal plans 42, 43, 49, 122, 211, 241-249

Mediterranean Diet 138, 141

metabolic syndrome 27, 75-79

monosodium glutamate (MSG) 32, 33, 126,

monounsaturated fats 141

N

nuts 22, 48, 50, 63, 84, 115-146, 158, 218, 241-248

O

obesity and weight gain 9, 27, 56, 76

oils 34, 139, 141-146

olive oil 43, 116-123, 140-146, 190, 242

omega-3 fats and omega-6 fats 141-146, 202, 220

organic foods 47, 97, 197-207

overeating 32, 36, 84, 139, 150

P

parties and celebrations 72, 123
polyunsaturated fats 141
portion size 62, 88, 89, 117, 138, 160
potatoes 61, 113, 117, 120, 149, 158, 188, 203, 238
processed foods 32-37, 47, 73, 138-155, 165, 204, 207

R

recipes 15, 48-49, 189
refined carbohydrates 161
restaurant 32, 53, 113-126, 138, 143, 189, 206, 217

S

salad dressing 32, 33
saturated fat 107, 140, 141, 202
stevia 104, 107, 152
supplements 142, 219-221
sweeteners, artificial 68, 86, 103-107, 149, 152-155, 205
sweet potatoes 61, 63, 113, 115, 188

T

trans fats 117, 142-146, 34, 113
triglyceride levels 59, 75, 140, 228
type 2 diabetes 172

U

unsaturated fats 141

V

vigorous exercise 93, 171-186

W

water 24, 33, 59, 88, 93, 96, 102-110
watermelon 61, 62, 203, 238
WHO (World Health Organization) 102, 148
Whole grains 35, 58, 61, 85, 86, 117, 132, 149, 153-162, 241
Willpower 78, 122, 168, 211

Y

Yo-yo eating 20, 22, 29

NOTES

1 "The IDF Consensus Worldwide Definition of the Metabolic Syndrome." International Diabetes Federation. 2006.

2 Ibid.

Principle 4: Learning to Take Control of What You Eat

3 Kessler, David A. *The End of Overeating: Taking Control of the Insatiable American Appetite*. Emmaus, PA: Rodale, 2009.

4 "What Do Food Labels Really Mean?" Cleveland Museum of Natural History. Accessed June 3, 2016. *http://www.gcbl.org/live/food/healthy-diet/what-do-food-labels-really-mean*

Principle 9: Learning about Other Hormones

5 Unlike type II diabetes, type I (also called juvenile diabetes) is characterized by the inability of pancreas to make enough insulin from birth and is not a consequence of bad eating, lifestyle habits, and belly fat accumulation.

6 Schellekens, H., T. G. Dinan, and J. F. Cryan. "Ghrelin at the Interface of Obesity and Reward." Vitamins and Hormones. Accessed April 03, 2018. *https://www.ncbi.nlm.nih.gov/pubmed/23374722.*

Egecioglu, Emil, Elisabet Jerlhag, Nicolas Salomé, Karolina P. Skibicka, David Haage, Mohammad Bohlooly-Y, Daniel Andersson, Mikael Bjursell, Daniel Perrissoud, Jörgen A. Engel, and Suzanne L. Dickson. "PRECLINICAL

STUDY: FULL ARTICLE: Ghrelin Increases Intake of Rewarding Food in Rodents." Addiction Biology. May 06, 2010. Accessed April 03, 2018. *https:// onlinelibrary.wiley.com/doi/full/10.1111/j.1369-1600.2010.00216.x.*

Principle 10: Understanding Metabolic Syndrome

7   "Just 'weight' until Menopause: How Estrogen Deficiency Affects Women's Fat Absorption." ScienceDaily. March 27, 2013. Accessed April 04, 2018. *https:// www.sciencedaily.com/releases/2013/03/130327144131.htm.*

   "Menopause and Weight Gain - HRT and Weight Gain." Weight Loss & Management for Women with BHRT | BodyLogicMD. Accessed April 04, 2018. https:// www.bodylogicmd.com/for-women/hormones-and-weight-gain.

8   *"The IDF Consensus Worldwide Definition of the Metabolic Syndrome." International Diabetes Federation. 2006. https://www.idf.org/webdata/docs/IDF_Meta_ def_final.pdf*

Step 1: Eat Less Every Meal

9   *Andrade, A.M., G. W. Greene, and K. J. Melanson. "Eating Slowly Led to Decreases in Energy Intake Within Meals in Healthy Women." July 2008. http://www. ncbi.nlm.nih.gov/pubmed/18589027.*

10 *MacDonald, Ann. "Why Eating Slowly May Help You Feel Full Faster." Harvard Health Blog. October 19, 2010. Accessed April 04, 2018. https://www.health.harvard.edu/blog/why-eating-slowly-may-help-you-feel-full-faster-20101019605.*

11 *http://merriam-webster.com. Accessed June 3, 2016*

Step 2: Moderate Exercise

12 *Tudor-Locke, Catrine, and David R. Bassett. "How Many Steps/Day Are Enough?" Sports Medicine 34, no. 1 (2004): 1-8.*

Step 3: Drinks

13 *Yang, Qing. The Yale Journal of Biology and Medicine. June 2010. Accessed April*

04, 2018. https://www.ncbi.nlm.nih.gov/pmc/articles/PMC2892765/.

14 *6. Fowler, Sharon P.G., Ken Williams, and Helen P. Hazuda. "Diet Soda Intake Is Associated with Long-Term Increases in Waist Circumference in a Biethnic Cohort of Older Adults: The San Antonio Longitudinal Study of Aging." Journal of the American Geriatrics Society J Am Geriatr Soc 63, no. 4 (2015): 708-15.*

15 *"Dehydration." Symptoms. Accessed February 01, 2016. http://www.mayoclinic. org/diseases-conditions/dehydration/basics/symptoms/con-20030056.*

Step 6: Fats

16 *http://www.webmd.com/diet/its-full-fat-and-helps-you-lose-weight?page=2*

17 *Simopoulos, A. P. "Importance of the Ratio of Omega-6/Omega-3 Essential Fatty Acids: Evolutionary Aspects." World Review of Nutrition and Dietetics Omega-6/ Omega-3 Essential Fatty Acid Ratio: The Scientific Evidence, 2003, 1-22.*

18 *"AHA's Recommendations on Omega-3 and Omega-6 Fats." Mercola.com. Accessed February 03, 2016. http://articles.mercola.com/sites/articles/archive/2012/01/12/ aha-position-on-omega-6-fats.aspx.*

Excess Omega 6 and Inflammation

19 *Patterson, E., R. Wall, G. F. Fitzgerald, R. P. Ross, and C. Stanton. "Health Implications of High Dietary Omega-6 Polyunsaturated Fatty Acids." Journal of Nutrition and Metabolism 2012 (2012): 1-16.*

20 *Cunnane, S. C., K. R. McAdoo, and D. F. Horrobin. "N-3 Essential Fatty Acids Decrease Weight Gain in Genetically Obese Mice." The British Journal of Nutrition. July 1986. Accessed April 04, 2018. https://www.ncbi.nlm.nih.gov/ pubmed/3676212/.*

21 *Hill, A. M., J. D. Buckley, K. J. Murphy, and P. R. Howe. "Combining Fish-oil Supplements with Regular Aerobic Exercise Improves Body Composition and Cardiovascular Disease Risk Factors." The American Journal of Clinical Nutrition. May 2007. Accessed April 04, 2018. https://www.ncbi.nlm.nih.gov/ pubmed/17490962.*

22 *Patterson, E., R. Wall, G. F. Fitzgerald, R. P. Ross, and C. Stanton. "Health Implications of High Dietary Omega-6 Polyunsaturated Fatty Acids." Journal of Nutrition and Metabolism 2012 (2012): 1-16.*

Step 7: Sugars

23 *"WHO Calls on Countries to Reduce Sugars Intake among Adults and Children."* *WHO. Accessed February 03, 2016. http://who.int/mediacentre/news/releases/2015/sugar-guideline/en/.*

24 *Kessler, David A. The End of Overeating: Taking Control of the Insatiable American Appetite. Emmaus, PA: Rodale, 2009.*

25 *Pollan, Michael. "When a Crop Becomes King." Accessed February 03, 2016. http://michaelpollan.com/articles-archive/when-a-crop-becomes-king/.*

26 *"U.S. Sugar Policy." SugarCane.org. Accessed February 03, 2016. http://sugarcane. org/global-policies/policies-in-the-united-states/sugar-in-the-united-states.*

27 *"Result Filters." National Center for Biotechnology Information. Accessed February 03, 2016. http://www.ncbi.nlm.nih.gov/pubmed/20086073.*

28 *"A Sweet Problem: Princeton Researchers Find That High-fructose Corn Syrup Prompts Considerably More Weight Gain." Princeton University. Accessed April 04, 2018. https://www.princeton.edu/news/2010/03/22/sweet-problem-princeton-researchers-find-high-fructose-corn-syrup-prompts.*

29 *"Can Fiber Protect Against Cancer?" WebMD. Accessed February 03, 2016. http:// www.webmd.com/diet/fiber-cancer.*

Step 9: Salt

30 *"Salt's Effects." Blood Pressure: On Your Body. Accessed February 04, 2016. http:// www.bloodpressureuk.org/microsites/salt/Home/Whysaltisbad/Saltseffect.*

31 *"Salt and Sodium." The Nutrition Source. Accessed February 04, 2016. http:// www.hsph.harvard.edu/nutritionsource/salt-and-sodium/.*

Step 10: Alcohol

32 *"Alcohol: Balancing Risks and Benefits." The Nutrition Source. Accessed February 04, 2016. http://www.hsph.harvard.edu/nutritionsource/alcohol-full-story/*

33 *"Health Benefits of Red Wine Antioxidant Questioned in Study" Medical News Today. Accessed February 04, 2016. http://www.medicalnewstoday.com/articles/276718.php*

34   *"Alcohol: Balancing Risks and Benefits." The Nutrition Source. Accessed February 04, 2016. http://www.hsph.harvard.edu/nutritionsource/alcohol-full-story/.*

Step 11: Vigorous Exercise

35   *"Aging Changes in Body Shape: MedlinePlus Medical Encyclopedia." U.S National Library of Medicine. Accessed February 04, 2016. https://www.nlm.nih.gov/medlineplus/ency/article/003998.htm.*

36   *"Result Filters." National Center for Biotechnology Information. Accessed February 04, 2016. http://www.ncbi.nlm.nih.gov/pubmed/8477683.*

37   *Boutcher, Stephen H. Journal of Obesity. 2011. Accessed April 04, 2018. https://www.ncbi.nlm.nih.gov/pmc/articles/PMC2991639/.*

Step 13: Sleep

38   *"What Happens When You Sleep?" National Sleep Foundation. Accessed February 05, 2016. https://sleepfoundation.org/how-sleep-works/what-happens-when-you-sleep.*

39   *"How Eating Carbs at Night Affects the Growth Hormone." LIVESTRONG. COM. 2015. Accessed February 05, 2016. http://www.livestrong.com/article/498071-how-eating-carbs-at-night-affects-the-growth-hormone/*

40   *"National Sleep Foundation Recommends New Sleep Times." National Sleep Foundation Recommends New Sleep Times. Accessed February 05, 2016. https://sleepfoundation.org/media-center/press-release/national-sleep-foundation-recommends-new-sleep-times.*

41   *"Lose Weight Before Trying Other Sleep Apnea Treatments." NPR. Accessed February 05, 2016. http://www.npr.org/sections/health-shots/2013/09/23/225429783/lose-weight-before-trying-cpap-sleep-apnea-treatments.*

Step 14: Go Organic

42   *"Organic.org—Organic FAQ." Organic.org. Accessed February 05, 2016. http://www.organic.org/home/faq.*

43   *"Organic Food Not Proven Healthier or Safer, Study Finds" Food Safety News. 2012. Accessed February 05, 2016. http://www.foodsafetynews.com/2012/09/organic-food-not-proven-healthier-or-safer-study-finds/#.VrUXgbIrLIV.*

44   *"Don't Eat Your Organic Veggies." New York Post 2013. Accessed February 06, 2016. http://nypost.com/2013/01/14/dont-eat-your-organic-veggies/.*

45   *"The Doctor Trying to Solve the Mystery of Food Allergies." NPR. Accessed February 07, 2016. http://www.npr.org/2013/04/15/177319365/the-doctor-trying-to-solve-the-mystery-of-food-allergies.*

46   *"Why Is Allergy Increasing?" Allergy UK. Accessed February 07, 2016. https:// www.allergyuk.org/why-is-allergy-increasing/why-is-allergy-increasing.*

47   *"40 Organizations That Are Shaking Up the Food System." Food Tank RSS. Accessed February 06, 2016. http://foodtank.com/news/2013/05/forty-organizations-that-are-shaking-up-the-food-system.*

48   *"Best Places to Buy Organic Foods Without Going Broke." http://www.kiplinger. com. Accessed February 06, 2016. http://www.kiplinger.com/article/spending/ T050-C011-S001-best-places-to-buy-organic-food-on-a-budget.html.*

49   *"Natural" on Food Labeling" http://www.fda.gov/Food/GuidanceRegulation/GuidanceDocumentsRegulatoryInformation/LabelingNutrition/ucm456090.htm*

50   *"Grass Fed Marketing Claim Standard." https://www.ams.usda.gov/grades-standards/beef/grassfed*

51   *"Fish Faceoff: Wild Salmon vs. Farmed Salmon—Health Essentials from Cleveland Clinic." Health Essentials from Cleveland Clinic. 2014. Accessed February 06, 2016. http://health.clevelandclinic.org/2014/03/fish-faceoff-wild-salmon-vs-farmed-salmon/*

52   *Holtcamp, Wendee. Environmental Health Perspectives. February 2012. Accessed April 04, 2018. https://www.ncbi.nlm.nih.gov/pmc/articles/PMC3279464/.*

Step 15: Be Happy for the Rest of Your Life

53   *Ryan, Richard M., N. Weinstein, J. Bernstein, K. W. Brown, L. Mistretta, and M. Gagné. "Vitalizing Effects of Being Outdoors and in Nature." Journal of Environmental Psychology 30, no. 2 (2010): 159-68.*

54   *"Spending Time in Nature Makes People Feel More Alive, Study Shows." Rochester News. Accessed February 07, 2016. http://www.rochester.edu/news/show. php?id=3639.*

55   *Cutler, Zach. "The 5 Benefits of Being Optimistic." Entrepreneur. May 14, 2015. Accessed April 06, 2018. https://www.entrepreneur.com/article/246204.*

56 *"How Much Calcium Do You Really Need? - Harvard Health." Harvard Health. Accessed February 07, 2016. http://www.health.harvard.edu/staying-healthy/how-much-calcium-do-you-really-need.*

57 *"Office of Dietary Supplements - Calcium." NIH Office of Dietary Supplements. Accessed April 06, 2018. https://ods.od.nih.gov/factsheets/Calcium-Consumer/.*

58 *"How Much Calcium Do You Really Need?" Harvard Health. Accessed February 07, 2016. http://www.health.harvard.edu/staying-healthy/how-much-calcium-do-you-really-need.*

59 *"The Risks of Excess Vitamins and Other Nutrients." WebMD. Accessed February 07, 2016. http://www.webmd.com/vitamins-and-supplements/nutrition-vitamins-11/fat-water-nutrient?page=1.*

60 *"Body Mass Index (BMI)." Encyclopedia of Public Health: 90. https://www.nhlbi.nih.gov/health/educational/lose_wt/BMI/bmi_tbl.pdf.*

61 *"The IDF Consensus Worldwide Definition of the Metabolic Syndrome." International Diabetes Federation. 2006. https://www.idf.org/webdata/docs/IDF_Meta_def_final.pdf.*

Appendix C: Exercise

62 *http://www.health.harvard.edu/diet-and-weight-loss/calories-burned-in-30-minutes-of-leisure-and-routine-activities*

Appendix D: List of Sugar Names

63 *"Learn to Recognize the 56 Different Names for Sugar." Institute for Responsible Nutrition. Accessed February 07, 2016. http://www.responsiblefoods.org/sugar_names.*

Made in the USA
Middletown, DE
29 January 2020